T0049939

LIFE,
DEATH
and *Biscuits*

LIFE,
DEATH
and Biscuits

ANTHEA ALLEN

HARPER
element

HarperElement
An imprint of HarperCollins*Publishers*
1 London Bridge Street
London SE1 9GF

www.harpercollins.co.uk

HarperCollins*Publishers*
Macken House, 39/40 Mayor Street Upper
Dublin 1, D01 C9W8, Ireland

First published by HarperElement 2022
This paperback edition published 2023

3 5 7 9 10 8 6 4 2

Text © Anthea Allen 2022

Photographs courtesy of the author with the following exceptions:
p5 (top) Lubo Ivanko/Getty Images; p5 (bottom) © BBC via
Getty Images

Anthea Allen asserts the moral right to
be identified as the author of this work

For my wonderful family who love me and
stand by me no matter what.

Elisabeth, my support, my partner, my safe
space, my love. Our life and devotion deeply
rooted together for over 30 years – my honest
and most constructive critic and biggest fan.

My extraordinary, brilliant and incredible
children, Claudia and Peter.

Ilaria, my adopted Italian eye-liner daughter
and kindred spirit.

'Nurses are beautiful, hilarious, tireless heroes.'

Claudia Gilbert-Allen, 2020

'This situation has united us all, in a way
that we still do not understand and for which
there is no word that defines it, but that
will always be there.'

Mónica De La Fuente Izquierdo, 2020

'The entire premise of Intensive Care Medicine
is purely built on and around the strength,
foundation, courage, versatility, extraordinary
skill, knowledge and humanity of our
Critical Care Nursing Cadre.'

Dr Jey Jeyanathan, 2021

CONTENTS

PROLOGUE

I am a Critical Care nurse, a senior sister at St George's University Hospitals NHS Trust in Tooting, south-west London. I am the lead for nurse recruitment for adult Critical Care. I am also a mum, partner, daughter, sister, friend, and I have a huge capacity to love.

Yet I am a nurse through to my bones. It was what I wanted to be 'when I grew up'. It was this job that connected me on such an incredible level with the superb team of nurses that I have the very great honour to work with. This team who united and fought through Covid – twice.

In March 2020 the Health Secretary, Matt Hancock, said on the BBC's evening news: 'As the peak of the coronavirus pandemic approaches we need more ventilators to fight Covid-19.' These were in short supply across the globe. Rolls-Royce, Dyson and other manufacturing firms were to make more ventilators, and the British government ordered hundreds of ventilators from China.

There was no mention of Critical Care nurses, who are skilled, trained and competent at safely using the ventilator, a complex piece of machinery. Not all doctors know how to programme a ventilator. It doesn't matter how many ventilators there are, Critical Care nurses are required to operate them. We don't have enough Critical Care nurses – they are what we need most.

Matt Hancock's statement, and simply wanting to do something for our amazing team, put me on the first step of a long road that would eventually become this book. And it all began with a request for biscuits.

I wrote one email, a plea for help. That was the beginning. I sent it to a group of local contacts, friends and neighbours, just asking for biscuits. The response was incredible. I ran out of words to say thank you, so I started to tell stories to explain the situation that we – the nurses on Critical Care at George's – found ourselves in.

Once a week I would send an email, and each time I was astonished by the response. My emails were forwarded and read by people who were in lockdown all over the world – I'd receive replies from Canada, New Zealand and South Africa. There was interest in the national media and celebrities, not to mention the floods of donations and incredible generosity from individuals and organisations desperate to help. People wanted to hear about what it was like on the front line, which was all the encouragement I needed to keep writing.

As the weeks and then months of the pandemic progressed, I was numbed by the ordeal of fighting the virus on the front line, and I felt a responsibility for our junior nurses. They were young and many were so far from home. Their fresh faces looked terrified. I remember being young and scared when I started working on Critical Care, and I wasn't sure how they were managing.

I, of course, want to protect their privacy in this book, but most of all I want to protect the privacy of the patients, who are vulnerable and place their trust in us. They have to do so and that must always be respected. All the stories you are about to read are true, but I have chopped and changed details so that no one can be identified. On occasion I have asked permission of the patients or their next of kin in order to include their names and their stories.

The doctors were phenomenal, but it is always about the doctors. This is a book about a family of nurses, Covid and love. I want you to be able to see what we saw. The extraordinary, the shocking, the impossible – the gory. The hideousness of injury and loss. The triumph over adversity and the little moments of amazing that are always just around the corner whenever nurses are involved. We get to see all the faces of humanity. Nothing makes sense and everything makes sense.

I hope in some way this book might help us to understand and to remember.

Anthea Allen, February 2022

In March 2020, when I wrote my first email requesting biscuits, I had no idea that my musings would become a book and, more shockingly, a *Sunday Times* bestseller.

Following the publication of *Life, Death and Biscuits* in February 2022, I received a handwritten letter of thanks from the Prince of Wales, now King Charles III. The Queen requested a copy of the book that you are about to read. I have received countless emails, letters and cards, including some from past patients, doctors, the parents of some of my colleagues and many from students and qualified nurses who thank me for sharing their story. As a result of writing this book, I am now asked to give talks about my experiences, and my audiences include the nurses who are newly recruited at St George's Hospital.

A story about nurses, love and Covid. It is possible to defy our expectations of ourselves, as I learnt when working through the pandemic. Looking back, it is almost as if it never happened – the unrelenting, horrific Covid-19 trenches just a period in time. We broke, we healed and we mostly reconstructed.

There are spaces within our hospital that still trigger memories and emotions. And those who worked together through the pandemic will always be united as our experience will be embedded within our hearts forever.

Anthea Allen, December 2022
@lifedeathbiscuits

HOW IT BEGAN

It was a Wednesday in early March 2020 when I returned to work. I had been in Dorset for a few days, staying with my parents. My father was taking his final church service as an Anglican priest after 63 years in the ministry (he was ordained at York Minster on my mother's twenty-first birthday). There were celebrations at their local parish church. My father led his last service, preached his last sermon and gave his last communion.

St Mary's is a Grade I listed building in Sturminster Newton, built in 1486. It's a quaint church with a carved wagon roof, glorious stained-glass windows and narrow wooden pews, with each person kneeling on an individually made hassock. The average age of the parishioners was about 70, it seemed, on a Sunday morning, but a little sectioned-off area with tiny wooden chairs and a display of children's illustrated Bibles and stories of Christian faith involving a family of squirrels said otherwise.

My parents' ginger cat waited outside, sitting on the stone wall as she did every Sunday, waiting patiently to walk them home. My father was cheered and toasted with

Prosecco and cake, and given a gift that all the local church-goers had contributed towards.

After a roast lunch at my parents' home, I drove back to London. LBC was on the radio in the car – more talk about coronavirus – but I didn't pay much attention. I connected my phone's playlist via Bluetooth and listened instead to Coldplay.

*   *   *

I have hundreds of stories to tell about what I've seen over the years. I remember the man who'd been driving too fast and wasn't wearing a seatbelt. A horse stepped into the road, the man braked and was catapulted out of the car and impaled on a wooden fence spike. I've nursed a woman who was 30 weeks pregnant when she fell off a balcony, a man injured in a boating accident, victims of road rage, sisters in a suicide pact, a woman who fell in front of a train, someone who had surgery to remove a chair leg from his rectum.

And I have nursed the regular sick and post-operative patients who come to us. Sepsis, ruptured bowel, respiratory failure, gastrointestinal bleed, broken bones, anaphylaxis; patients undergoing complex surgery or those who have underlying health issues that may affect their current condition or surgery. Asthma, diabetic problems, fitting, overdose, ruptured spleen, all manner of injury and illness, from the bizarre to the ridiculous – and sometimes the mundane.

There has been tragedy, pain, recovery, rehabilitation and devastation, but I have also seen individuals pull through against all odds, healing and surviving. I have seen and experienced some incredible and wonderful things. Nothing is predictable. That's how it is.

I have witnessed the horrors of what people do to each other. The serious acts of violence. A man who had been tied up or held down and had his fingers cut off (particularly striking because of the meticulous way in which the amputation had been executed). I have seen desperately sad situations: a whole family killed except for the three-year-old child whose future, in an instant, was altered unimaginably. I have witnessed life and death in the extreme.

After more than 20 years of working in Critical Care, I really did think that I had seen everything. But I was wrong. After my time off work spent visiting my parents, I returned for my first shift. That was when I realised that Covid was real and it was here, in St George's Hospital, in Tooting, south-west London.

Outside, it was quiet. Much of the hospital had been emptied and the drama was confined behind the doors of Critical Care. There was an eerie stillness as I walked into work. Our team were already immersed in the extraordinary; until you are there, it is impossible to imagine. As the effects of the pandemic increased, so too would the amount of space required within the hospital to deal with the incoming patients. More hospitalisations meant more beds were required. It had all begun, in my absence, with Covid-positive patients being admitted one after the other after the other. This was unprecedented. This was the beginning of something quite unimaginable.

In the Atkinson Morley Wing of the hospital, I got my first glimpse of the effects of Covid. There was tension in the air. I started working on Brodie Ward, a neurosurgical ward. Its regular patients decanted elsewhere, the ward had now morphed into an Intensive Care Unit (ICU), but this was not an environment in which to nurse a critically ill patient.

The unit had been divided into 'pods', each one holding five or six patients. The pods were like glass bubbles with sealed doors, and there were lines taped on the floor to mark the boundaries separating the safe zones from the unsafe zones. You could only step over a line if you were wearing full PPE (Personal Protective Equipment).

Many other parts of the hospital had been closed, thereby preventing the spread of coronavirus. Elective surgery had stopped; clinic work had stopped. All routine procedures had stopped. The hospital was forced to grind to a halt for safety reasons. Suddenly everything was different. Everything had changed.

A group of nurses had been formed to help fight the disease. Nurses and doctors from the other units had been drafted in to work with us in Critical Care. Plenty of them had volunteered – and there were also nurses who had retired, were doing something different or whose professional registration had lapsed. We needed all nurses, any nurse, but mostly we needed Critical Care nurses. (Later we also had men and women from the army drafted in to help and support us.)

However, very few of them saw death as frequently as the Critical Care nurses. Many of them had never seen death at all. They were willing to give their all, but usually they worked in departments where patients were not seriously ill and where deadly infection was not a concern. Some nurses came from the maxillofacial unit, specialising in facial and oral surgery. When they were asked how they could help the coronavirus patients, one of the nurses replied half-jokingly, 'We can sort out their teeth.'

*   *   *

'Can I work with you?' said an Indian nurse I knew well. She'd be my co-worker for that first day in one of the pods. I knew that her husband and son were in India; we didn't know it then, but it would be a year before they were able to return. There was another Critical Care nurse in charge and, while I knew her, I had never worked with her, as she worked on a different unit.

That first day was also an introduction to wearing PPE the entire shift. We had received lessons on donning and doffing, during which we wore the PPE for five minutes. The PPE was essential and was also highly controversial because the media was informing us that the NHS was running out of supplies. The government hadn't ordered enough to cope with the demand.

Our PPE was a gown, face mask covering our mouth and nose, and a visor. We would cover our head with a J Cloth-style theatre cap. The PPE was cumbersome and uncomfortable, and the mask made it difficult to breathe. Once we were in PPE, we were incredibly hot and anonymous. (In those early days we were identifiable only by our eyes. Later we wrote our names on sticky name labels. I designed them in my head during a bout of insomnia, and CriticalNhs sourced a printer and delivered rolls and rolls of the different-coloured sticky labels, which denoted our job title and name.)

We worked in a pod with another nurse, who was a conscript from endoscopy. We didn't know her or even what she was able to do. Together, the three of us looked after five Covid-positive patients. That first day was a pool of tension and my memories of it are blurred and hazy, set against the backdrop of the blue-grey walls of the ward. Soon these colours would come to dominate my dreams at night.

The oxygen supply wasn't working at one of the bed spaces: the white hose at the back of the ventilator kept jumping out of the oxygen port in the wall, which caused the ventilator to sound its alarm and the patient's ventilation to be disrupted. We would have to move the patient to a bed space where there was a fully functioning oxygen supply. I ordered several large oxygen cylinders and the nurse in charge of the shift reported the issue. We could not leave the bed space unoccupied, however, despite the broken oxygen port, as we needed all space available. We had to admit another patient who required non-invasive ventilation (NIV) and was deteriorating on the ward. We would deliver her oxygen from a massive cylinder next to her bed until the broken port was fixed. Yet more tubing and equipment to take up the limited space we were working in.

I realised at that moment how we took for granted our purpose-built Critical Care. Moving the bed was planned like a regimented procedure, as there were only three of us and the patient was sick and unstable. Meanwhile, another patient was pulling at his tracheostomy, trying to remove it, too ill to be aware that it was helping him to live. And another patient was trying to get out of bed.

We were in an impossible situation that we needed to manage the best way we could. Usually, I would have other senior staff to discuss this with, but we had to move the patient urgently, safely and quickly, using the people and resources we had available at that moment. The move of only about 12 metres went smoothly. We bagged the patient (manual breaths delivering oxygen) while pushing the bed and haemofiltration machine, drip poles and pumps. The cardiac monitor was balanced on the bed.

Doctors hovered slightly beyond the taped boundary doorway, issuing requests and instructions. In the early days doctors did not come into the bays unless required to perform a procedure or examine a patient. The less traffic the better, in an attempt to keep Covid contained.

One consultant suggested we use walkie-talkies as a way of sharing information but avoiding staff entering or leaving the bays unnecessarily.

We also discussed having a visual list of items most used, and when nurses needed something we'd point to it on a chart through the glass window and the runner on standby outside the bay could find and deliver whatever drug/tube/gadget/liquid we needed.

We were too busy getting on with the process of looking after our patients, so these things never happened.

*   *   *

What were we dealing with? What weapons were being deployed by Covid, the invisible enemy?

People presented at hospital with flu, or with what might seem like a cold or cough, but they were struggling to breathe. To put it in perspective, a healthy person takes approximately 12 to 16 breaths every minute, while many of the coronavirus patients were gasping on 35 to 40 breaths per minute.

We took arterial blood gases – a test to measure the acidity of the blood and the levels of oxygen and carbon dioxide. When a person is struggling to breathe, the carbon dioxide level is usually quite high. The effort to breathe was immense: their respiratory rate would increase, as would their heart rate, the body putting in a monumental effort to supply the cells with the oxygen it so desperately required. The patients became exhausted and had severe respiratory failure. This can place the heart under enormous pressure – imagine running up a never-ending hill.

We gave drugs to sedate the coronavirus patients struggling for breath, and then we intubated them (put a breathing tube down their throat). The tube was attached to a ventilator, which expands the patient's lungs and increases oxygenation, so that the patient does not have to breathe for themselves.

As humans, we breathe through negative pressure: we suck in air, or inhale, and it is drawn into our lungs. The ventilator, however, is positive pressure: it's pushing air into the lungs at a set volume or pressure. This different way of breathing increases the intrathoracic pressure which, in turn, can cause other problems. Often when somebody requires intubation in the critical care setting, both the heart and lungs are at the point of exhaustion and start to fail. It is almost as if the body heaves a huge sigh of exhaustion and gives up.

The lungs of some patients were swollen and bleeding. Many Covid patients suffered from blood clots, and their blood pressure would start to fail. They were on drugs to increase blood pressure, and this led to vasoconstriction: the blood vessels tighten to reduce the surface volume within the veins and arteries and so push up the blood pressure. (It has been suggested that Covid is not necessarily a respiratory problem, but a multifaceted, nasty disease which also causes problems with clotting, including clots within the lungs creating further difficulties with breathing.) With Covid, we would discover, nothing was straightforward.

There is, by the way, no such thing as a 'life-support machine'. This is a layman's term. There is cardiac support for cardiac failure, and it amounts to drugs or a balloon pump. The pump helps a failing heart to support the blood pressure. Renal support is filtration or dialysis, while respiratory support includes support with breathing, possibly requiring a ventilator and oxygen. A coma is a state of prolonged unconsciousness, either induced by medicine or as a result of brain injury or due to a stroke. Coma can also be the result of brain infection or encephalitis.

*   *   *

And then there were the deaths on that first day. The ones that I witnessed. When there was no more we could do for one of the patients and he sadly died, I was overwhelmed by the reality that these people were dying and they were on their own. It was extraordinarily sad, and suddenly I felt like I couldn't breathe. It was so hot.

'Go to the window,' said my colleague. 'Just go to the window. Open the window and lean out.' I looked at the nurse and saw only her eyes. I had years more experience than her, but she had more experience of working in the insufferable conditions of the coronavirus unit. 'That's what I do,' she said.

She was right. I stood for a moment or two with my head out of the window and my back to the ward, and I breathed and breathed again. Then a man went into cardiac arrest and I flipped back – in an instant, I got my head together, ready to deal with the action. Another death.

And then someone came into the room, another unidentifiable person in a hazmat suit. 'We've got two more coming in,' she said. 'We'll put one here' – and she pointed to a space by the window. 'And we'll put another one there.' She jabbed a finger towards another space for a bed. 'And can you move those bodies?'

I thought to myself, *But I haven't got a bed.* The other nurse nodded towards the bodies and the two new arrivals. She said, 'Those two are dead. These ones are alive. We have to think like that.' Again, she was right.

I went for a break, and when I came back I panicked. The bodies of the two men were on beds, pushed up against a wall together to make way for the new arrivals. For a split second I thought that the men had been mixed up; they both looked the same. It was so busy it was impossible to get to know a patient. Usually I would know my patient's name – but not now.

My God, which is which? Who is who? I hadn't mixed them up, thankfully. There was a name tag on the ankle of one of the men. Usually we are meticulous, putting two name tags on each patient. Now, consumed by the frantic pace, it felt as if we were having to cut corners and deviate from usual policy.

When a patient dies there is a protocol, but even that had changed. The porters collect a body once they are wrapped and in a body bag and the paperwork completed, but at the beginning the porters were terrified and would not even enter the ward. We had to wheel the bed out of the pod to the door, where the porters would collect them and transfer the body to the mortuary.

At times I felt helpless. I *was* helpless. Later, when people asked about it, I'd say, 'It was like I was sitting in an armchair watching my house burn down.'

*   *   *

I do remember one evening – whether it was the first, the second or third, I'm not sure – when the shift had ended, and I removed my visor, mask, gown and cap. I walked along the corridor in a trance and went to our changing room. 'Have you got a moment?' said one of the young nurses, poking her head round the door.

'Of course, yeah. Sit down.' She sat, and then a few seconds later she burst into tears. I put my arms around her. As I would see in the subsequent days, weeks and months, when the young nurses cried, they did so as if they were children, burying their heads into my neck. There would be times when I'd realise my ears and neck were wet with their tears.

Each of them was mentally battered by the experience, just as you would expect. One nurse, in her early twenties, would say to me a couple of months later, 'I was never worried for myself. Maybe I didn't think much about it. But we were young, working hard and trying to do our best. I never told my mum that I was working with Covid patients. She's my mum so really she should have known, but I never told her.'

These kids – the young nurses – were on their own. Some of them had come from other countries to work in Britain. They had left behind their mothers, fathers, siblings and friends. English might not have been their first language. Covid would bring death and destruction, but it would also be the strange but unbreakably strong bond that united the nurses in Critical Care.

Odd though it sounds, that hospital was to become the place where I felt most at home. Many other nurses felt the same way. I wanted to be there, and I would go there on my day off. I wanted to be alongside the other nurses. As one nurse would say, 'The situation has united us in a way which we still don't understand, and there is no way to define it, but it will always be there.'

I felt guilty if I was not at work. My colleagues were struggling. We set up and prepared new areas for Covid patients. A few days earlier what had seemed like a ghost town – the empty shell of a ward as it was made ready for new arrivals – now heaved with doctors and nurses in PPE as they tried to cope with yet more arrivals. The Trust were discussing the next area of the hospital that could be claimed and transformed into a coronavirus ICU. The wards were busy, having lost many of their staff, who were transferred to Critical Care. Student nurses were now expected to work as trained nurses and as many agency staff as possible were employed. This was unreal, unsustainable, unimaginable and … there are not even the words.

I was working alongside a doctor who had served in the army. 'This is worse than Afghanistan,' he said to me. 'In Afghanistan we were prepared. The injuries were visible, the whole thing was visual. With this, everything seems invisible. We've got patients who are dying, but there are no wounds, no blood. We're trying to protect ourselves against this but don't really know how to. It's the unseen enemy. We're not trained for this. We're not prepared. It's shocking and it's affecting not just us but the whole world.'

*　　*　　*

I pride myself on my end-of-life care. Usually families stay with their dying relative. They'll hold their hand, talk to them. They lie next to them or brush their hair. But families being present when a loved one died came to an abrupt end. Families were not allowed to visit. The desperately sad reality was that patients died without their loved ones there. Nurses were with them instead.

Often during the pandemic, but not always, family were united with the patient via modern technology to say their last farewell. We had been given iPads which had been reconfigured by the IT department and were supposed to be simple to use, with a sort of one-click easiness. To me, the process seemed more like 17 clicks. I couldn't work it out, and I wasn't the only one. And that was assuming you could even find one. When you finally did, often it had not been charged, revealing 13 per cent battery power.

One Covid patient was a woman in her late forties. A couple of weeks before, she had been at a conference in New York. She thought she had a cold and became really unwell on the flight home. She'd competed in triathlons before, then the invisible enemy put her in here. Now she was dying, rapidly falling apart in front of me.

'Mummy, don't die! Don't die!' The screams from her twin daughters left a temporary tinnitus in my ear as I wedged the iPad near her face. It was a terrible situation, and then I heard the crinkling of a hazmat suit behind me.

'Are you a doctor?' I asked.

'No, I'm a priest.' He'd come in PPE to say some prayers.

I said to the daughters, 'There's a priest here. Would you like him to say a prayer?'

And the voices, distraught, said, 'Yes, please.'

*   *   *

Nurses deal with so much. Smelly feet, urine and blood. Being shouted at, being sworn at. I have removed tampons and contact lenses, sat on the floor with a wailing firefighter, transferred patients in an ambulance, transported live organs in a Learjet, picked out a denture from a bowl of vomit. Cleaned fungating tumours. Photographed tattoos on a body. I've coerced a confused patient back into bed, chased a paranoid, bleeding, naked patient down a corridor. Mopped up tears and poo. Hugged strangers. Delivered babies. Had a patient corner and threaten me. I've been a witness for a marriage. Cleaned up a puddle of diarrhoea, picked bags of cocaine out of faeces.

I have deloused a man, cleaned a maggot-infested tumour and applied leaches to an anal wound. Sung happy birthday to a patient, danced with a patient, been kicked and spat at. I have searched for a person's property, bought a patient a cappuccino, laughed until I ached, and washed and wrapped literally hundreds of dead bodies. We have an elastic job description! And now Covid ...

As new patients arrived, the burden became heavier on the staff. We got through 12-hours shifts, managing on two short breaks a day. Toilet breaks were also restricted and intermittent, partly because we didn't have time to go to the loo, and also because they required the removal of protective clothing followed by a change into new clothing. We were an exhausted, thirsty regiment of nurses. We ate on the hop, grabbing a bite of this, a bite of that, a sandwich here, a biscuit there. Some shops within the hospital now refused to serve staff in uniforms or scrubs, so on top of the sleep deprivation and dehydration, there was hunger too.

We were dealing with damage control, fire-fighting. The day was one long emergency and then it was the next day, and it kept going. No one in the entire hospital knew what the best thing was to do. We wore PPE in the Covid areas but nowhere else. Mask wearing was not a thing at that time.

One night, not long after my first shift in the Covid pods, when things were getting far worse, I returned home from work. It was 16 March, a Monday. I showered and poured myself a glass of wine. I felt the need to do something, anything, and although I care about the patients, I care about our nurses. I have always said that if you care for the nurses, they will care for the patients.

I sat at my laptop and typed an email to send to a few friends and the local community. I have lived in the area for 20 years. I have email addresses for parents at the schools that my children had attended, the PTA, contacts from swimming, football and ballet clubs, our neighbours from a street party, my Pilates group. I wanted to email any non-medical and local contacts that I had.

As many of you know, I am a senior sister on Critical Care. The hospital is in crisis – our executive staff are being amazing and the frontline staff incredible. My nursing colleagues expose themselves daily to the threat of Covid-19.

The hospital is doing all it can to protect the staff with PPE training to safely care for all patients.

We are opening other areas within the hospital to nurse critically ill patients and employing agency staff to help out.

We continue to receive trauma patients and those suffering from other medical issues through accident, illness or surgery.

I am proud of my colleagues. The nurses are stretched to the limit anyway but are now under immense pressure. I have seen tears, fear and exhaustion, and last week some of the shops within the hospital refused to sell food, drinks and snacks to staff in scrubs or uniforms, so staff missed meals. Supplies have been stolen and the hospital are working hard to put additional measures in place.

Please remember to spare a thought for the nurses who directly care for the patients and families on Critical Care and the dedicated wards in very difficult circumstances, frequently without appreciation: working long hours, skipping breaks and going the extra mile to ensure patients feel safe and well cared for. All while wearing cumbersome protective gear.

On Friday a friend of mine delivered a huge box of dough-nuts for the nurses on my unit that I took to work. They were so appreciated and within an hour were gone!

If you would like to do something for the nurses at your local hospital, please feel free to drop off a box of biscuits or something the staff can snack on with me or at the hospital, or at your local hospital marked for the nurses.

Please note: It doesn't matter how many ventilators are made; we need the skilled Critical Care nurses to operate them. Most doctors cannot operate a ventilator as it is not a skill required by a dermatologist, oncologist or surgeon who are brilliant within their own specialities, but we are all now stretched beyond the barriers of our performance.

Keep safe, wash your hands and remember – nurses are amazing.

Thank you.

I pressed send. At 9.06 – the moment I sent the email – I had no idea about what was to follow. I was prompted to ask for something sweet by an image that stays with me: I had seen a nurse stuff a doughnut in her mouth while on a quick toilet break, sugar all down her top, jam on her nose. She was laughing. It was a moment of normal that took place in an otherwise extraordinary situation. I only sent the email to get a box or two of chocolate brownies. I just wanted to do something, anything, to help and support our staff. The following day my doorstep was piled high with boxes of chocolates, cakes and biscuits.

Nor did I envisage that this would prompt me to begin a diary made up of my emails, a chronology of Covid on the front line. Through the emails that follow, I discovered an outlet. I found a way to voice the experience, to share the problems and burdens of this extraordinary ordeal. And for me personally, it became a form of therapy, a cathartic unburdening of my own struggle through the pandemic.

A friend would later say, 'It's just your word vomit, written down on paper.'

'No paper,' I said. 'I use my laptop!'

MARCH 2020

22 March

To all my friends, friends of friends, neighbours and this community.

I have been overwhelmed and amazed by the incredible generosity shown to my colleagues and myself since I sent my first email. I had hoped to gain some biscuits and possibly a homemade cake to share with my colleagues.

BUT ... I did not expect this response.

The support has been beyond incredible. I have so far received a total of nine bin bags packed with biscuits, chocolate, cake and cereal bars. My staff have been fed with pizza, curry, Mediterranean fare, homemade cookies and brownies, homemade bread, cheese, doughnuts and huge baskets of fresh fruit.

I have received cards, emails and messages of support.

Friends have given me a lift to work. Each day there is more. Last night I arrived home beyond exhausted and there was a tin of homemade shortbread sitting on the doorstep, with a card saying, 'Thank you, nurses.' I have no idea who made them, but thank you.

The local school has emailed me, offering support and to arrange food deliveries of sandwiches. The kindness of strangers, the warm spirit of local people and my very dear friends, as well as those further afield, has warmed my heart. Local friends have set up a funding page which has raised over £7,000 in two days. I have no words to express my gratitude.

The staff of Critical Care who are working tirelessly have been kept afloat by this support. They no longer have to bring their meals to work. We have shared food with the wards who are also caring for Covid patients.

We are all trained and competent in strict infection control procedure and the 'donning and doffing' of PPE. We are trained to care for Covid patients who are strictly cohorted together, supported by ward nurses and student nurses. The team of doctors, nurses, physiotherapists and other health-care professionals are working long hours with these patients, and we also have our usual non-Covid critically ill patients.

The entire Trust are being incredible. Doctors, nurses, reception staff, ward clerks, porters, cleaners, security, nurse educators, technicians, lab workers, blood bank staff, pharmacists, dietitians and many others who help in keeping the big ship St George's afloat.

I am proud to work for our NHS and please do not underestimate how much your kindness and generosity means to us all. As one nurse said, 'We are like the band in the *Titanic* film – we keep on playing while the ship goes down ...'

This ship will not sink and we will keep on keeping on.

Thank you, thank you, thank you.

Stay at home, wash your hands and be kind to each other.

Staff are working hard and are greatly affected emotionally by this crisis, but I have seen much laughing and chatting among my colleagues while they are munching on pizza!

Thank you, from the bottom of my heart.

*   *   *

I am a parent. We have two children. My son is at school and Claudia, my daughter, is a student at the University of Bristol. She took part in a dance show, and almost as soon as the curtain came down, the students were told that university lectures were cancelled for the foreseeable future. There were the first reported cases of Covid-19 in Bristol. The Friday show had to be cancelled as a member of the cast had come into contact with someone who had Covid. The show went ahead on the Saturday, however, as the theatre had been deep cleaned.

As lockdown loomed, Claudia had phoned and said, 'I want to come home.'

'When?'

'Can you come and get me tomorrow? I just feel that I want to be home.'

The following morning I drove from London to Bristol to collect her. Once Claudia was in the car, I suggested we go for a bite to eat. There were some restaurants that were still open. (Not for much longer, though: in a matter of days they'd all be closed.)

But no, Claudia was insistent: 'I just want to get home.'

As we drove, she seemed anxious about the coming months. 'What am I going to do until September? I can't go out. We can't see anybody. What am I going to do? I've got one essay to write.' Then a pause, and she added, 'I'm going to go crazy.'

24 March

Jonathan Silver is the Head of Clinical Engineering at St George's. He's responsible for the management of medical devices across the Trust – evaluating and buying them, advising on their use, investigating adverse incidents, ensuring staff are trained. He's posted on Facebook: 'Been ordered to take a day off today to prevent burnout, having spent eight long days straight at work doing everything possible to prepare for the onslaught of up to 600 critically ill patients to our 60-bed intensive care service.

'One thing is clear: we are a facing a situation close to battlefield medicine. We are forced to dispense with our usually very high standards of care, safety and dignity in order to give the masses a chance to survive.'

APRIL 2020

5 April

The ongoing support that overwhelmed me when I first made a request for biscuits has continued. @CriticalNhs has been set up and is run like a business – an efficient, well-run, immediate-response business started by my incredible friends who, in response to my initial email, also wanted to support and help.

This has exploded. I think you guys should run the NHS!

We needed biscuits, and from that came delicious meals three times a day for the Critical Care team and other areas of the hospital. We have PPE top-ups, fresh fruit and veg, spaghetti – scooped up fast by our Italian nurses – radios, chocolate, bespoke name badges, cake, hand cream, free parking at the hospital for staff, tablets for the patients to communicate with – and one night, fresh green leaves were delivered for the rabbit belonging to one of our nurses.

The compassion shown has been outstanding. The clapping, the rainbows and, for me, I appreciate every single email, text and message of support and the gifts and donations for our team that end up on my doorstep.

I have been a nurse for 25 years – 23 of those in Critical Care – and I thought I had seen everything. Critical Care has changed overnight. It's like being in a sci-fi movie: staff gowned up with visors, masks and head covers. Our usual capacity of ventilated beds has increased into wards, operating theatres and anaesthetic rooms. From three Critical Care units with a total of 66 beds, we now have 147 Critical Care beds in seven areas. Highly trained nurses who usually care for one intensive-care patient now have three to four patients, with helpers who are ward nurses; many have never before set foot on an intensive-care unit. It's a different environment, in a different world. This is before we escalate into ExCel, the exhibition centre in London's Docklands being set up as a hospital for Covid patients. How will this be staffed?

It's tough. It's claustrophobic in the gowns, masks and visors. Nurses are thirsty, enclosed in a room for 12 hours with the only escape coming when it's time to eat or visit the toilet. I saw one of my colleagues with blood on her scrubs, as she had no time to change her tampon. I went into the toilet in the bay to help her. I handed her new scrubs to change into, gave her a new tampon and helped her wash. It was not OK to put this young nurse in this position – she felt undignified – but it also was OK, as it didn't really matter at all – to me; we are friends and I just wanted to help her feel better and she trusted me.

It's raw and real. A halloumi wrap, pizza, curry or chocolate brownie is helping us through this tsunami.

I speak on behalf of nurses, as I am one. But we could not survive without doctors, porters, clerical staff, technicians, physios, dietitians, pharmacists, cleaners, mortuary team, lab staff, engineers, security and the fabulous volunteers whose step count exceeds 20,000 a day. Last week, one nurse notched up 27,000 steps in a day – the equivalent of about 11 miles.

The NHS staff work tirelessly, abandoning their days off and giving all that they have. We also have our usual Critical Care patients. Accidents, illness, cardiac arrests still happen, and people still stab and harm each other despite the world being in crisis.

I have mopped up tears and cuddled nurses and passed chocolate around – there is limited social distancing in the hospital. Many of our nurses are from Europe or Ireland and miss their families. A part of my usual role is nurse recruitment. I get to know the nurses well and the younger ones call me 'Mama Anthea'. I have become a temporary parent to some of our young nurses. One of the nurses calls me Mommy, which makes me proud and happy. It is now strange if she calls me Anthea.

*   *   *

Anyone who has ever visited a hospital will have noticed the incessant ringing of the telephones at the reception desks of wards and units. Perhaps you have tried to call but your call was never answered. The phones are answered, it's just that there are lots of phones that ring and lots of people who call.

Often it is the ward clerk who answers the phone, and sorts out other issues such as broken photocopiers, transfers notes from one place to another, orders items, books transport, ensures staff have access to our scrub dispenser, reports a broken light or adds patient details on the iClip IT system that we use. It's a job for a practical, hardworking, friendly person who can use their initiative and support our struggling team.

One of our ward clerks had just left and hadn't been replaced, and our matron said, 'I can't cope with the non-stop phones. Does anybody know someone sensible who could come in and work here?'

I said, 'What about Claudia? I picked her up from uni and she's at home, feeling bored.'

She said, 'Would she answer the phones?'

'She'd be brilliant.'

'Get her in, get her in ...'

I rang Claudia. I said, 'Would you like to work here?

'When will I start?'

'Tomorrow,' I said.

Claudia was at the hospital the following morning. We showed her round and hired her. Eight days after taking a bow on stage in Bristol, Claudia began as a ward clerk. It was a Monday, the eve of the tipping point of coronavirus. Ordinarily, she would have gone for an induction day, learning how to use the computers and answer the phones. Instead, she sat with one of our very experienced ward clerks on the reception desk, watching and learning as she went along. They clicked.

There are three phones and they ring in synchrony. 'Go ahead and answer,' she said to Claudia, and my daughter just cracked on with it. She had been in the job for 15 minutes. In at the deep end. On a floor above her, a coronavirus unit was being set up. (This would be the third, and the largest intensive treatment unit.) Claudia helped set it up and continually expanded her rather unusual job description. It was all hands on deck – normal did not apply anymore.

The new unit was a long corridor with bays coming off it. The patients who'd once occupied this area had now been cleared – either sent home or to wards in other parts of the hospital – and the entire ward had been scrubbed clean. Trollies of linen were wheeled in, and then Claudia and a few others set to work, making beds.

*   *   *

Thank you for caring for us. We will keep on keeping on. The 'keep calm and carry on' slogan from the 1940s rings true.

Keep clapping, put rainbows in your window and stay at home.

My thanks on behalf of a truly fabulous group of people – NURSES!

'All shall be well, and all shall be well, and all
manner of things shall be well.'

Julian of Norwich, fourteenth-century mystic

12 April

I have always been a chatty person. It takes a lot to take my
breath away. There are no words to describe the scenes and
way of working within our forever-expanding Critical Care.

ICU nurses are meticulous. Attention to detail is high on
our list. I have many friends who carefully label the jars in their
larders, as we are so conditioned to labelling drugs and equipment to ensure that we are alert to expiry dates or what a
specific drug is and its dose. ICU nurses love to label.

We keep a diary for patients. This is so that when they
recover they can know their journey. If they don't survive,
feedback tells us that these diaries are a comfort to the families. We brush patients' teeth; we change their position, the
way they are lying in bed. We talk to patients who are unconscious. We explain to family. We wash hair. We smuggle in a
dog to visit; we put a favourite teddy in the bed. We respect
religion, race, sexuality. I have repositioned a bed to face
Mecca and dropped off a Valentine card for an elderly patient's
wife.

We give the same high standard of skilled care to every
person. We deal with all intimate procedures for our patients,
as well as operating ventilators and supporting organ failure
with specialised drugs and machinery. We are a competent,

skilled, highly knowledgeable, kind, caring group of individuals who are proud to be Critical Care nurses.

It's different now. We are in a growing storm. We just fire-fight to do whatever we can to keep someone alive, try our best to help them beat this unrelenting deadly virus. We have nurses to help who are unfamiliar with the ICU environment. The personal care is impossible. One nurse said to me, 'I don't even know my patients' names.'

This is not our usual place of work. There is a backdrop. It's like being in a weird dream. We all have trouble sleeping and so many of our permanent nurses – they come from all over the world – want to go home. They probably will after this is done. We are broken.

True to form, there is hilarity amid the madness. Nurses have a sick sense of humour. We are laughing and crying and supporting each other. We have offers of counselling but the nurses are too busy and their priority outside the environment is to eat, sleep and have a very long shower. One day some of the nurses had the names of pop stars written on their gowns, rather than their own names. I didn't recognise Beyoncé at all – a large male cardiac ICU nurse, I think.

We feel wretched and exhausted and tired while at work. We feel guilty when not at work, as we know there are not enough staff with the patients. Nurses work extra days. If I am not at work, I am coordinating staffing, rushing through temporary staff, arranging ID cards and PC access, ordering supplies, plan-ning the opening of new makeshift areas and procuring new equipment, as well as talking to overwhelmed nurses.

I walked through one of the ICUs a few days ago and blew kisses at the nurses I know beneath swathes of fabric, plastic and paper. Possibly I didn't know them, but they got a kiss anyway. Today I received a text message from one of the Italian nurses: 'Please come by and send me flying kisses again.'

I once asked this Italian nurse what had inspired her to become a nurse. 'In a way, my father,' she replied. 'He passed away when I was quite young. Eleven. And I think in my mind, I wanted to be a nurse. Then I could look after people because I had not been able to look after him.' She graduated as a nurse in 2014, came to England a few years ago and, after 18 months, she came to St George's ICU. 'I'd heard that St George's was really good and I wanted to work in a trauma centre and do a little bit of intensive care,' she said. Three years later, she is still here, in the midst of this pandemic and probably feeling a million miles from Milan.

The level of anxiety increases immeasurably each day. It's often too traumatic and surreal to talk about what we see and do. It's particularly tough for the junior staff who work day after day, and are expected to suddenly lead and guide staff from other areas.

We live a parallel life while others take the quarantine art challenge, plan Easter egg hunts and are bored at home. We continue on and on and on, and still more patients arrive. They feel ill and scared. One man said, 'Please don't let me die.'

Thank you for your support. Keep it going. I think nurses will need support way beyond this time. Every card, email, text, WhatsApp makes a difference. The support I receive powers me on to support our incredible team of Critical Care nurses. If you know a nurse, send them a message or drop something on their doorstep.

This is a different way of nursing. Unchartered, with no end in sight.

There are many NHS workers, some unseen, who are struggling. The mortuary staff have an endless stream of dead bodies to store. Our mortuary is full. The lab technicians have to process the stream of swabs, as well as their daily testing of blood and specimens. Our technicians service, clean and calibrate the ventilators. At the beginning of the pandemic some of the machines we need to use are over 50 years old and repurposed. We use anaesthetic machines, designed for ventilating a patient during surgery. The pharmacy keeps up with the supply of drugs required. Recruitment are processing new, redeployed and temporary staff. Many NHS workers, the nurses and doctors on the front line and our entire team – I share your donations and messages with them too.

A junior doctor told me, 'When this is done – so am I. No amount of money could make me stay.' Then she asked, 'Who sent in the delicious figs?'

I appreciate all the messages. I can't always reply, as I am working or don't know what to say. Or it is just that I am totally exhausted.

Keep safe, keep smiling and never underestimate the importance of staying at home at this time.

*   *   *

Claudia was asked by a friend, 'Are any of the doctors hot?' Thanks to the PPE, the doctors' eyes are the only visible body parts. Claudia has other things on her mind, however. Her description of the smells of the Covid Critical Care: 'The smell of orange wipes, bleach and poo.'

After a day of bed-making, Claudia worked on the Tuesday and then she had a day off on Wednesday. When she returned to work on Thursday, she was stunned to discover that the bay where she had made up the beds just a couple of days earlier was now full with Covid-19 sufferers. The unit, which a few days earlier had seemed like a ghost town, was now heaving with staff in hazmat suits and PPE as they tried to cope with the new arrivals. The Trust were discussing the next part of the wing which could be claimed and transformed into a coronavirus unit.

'It was like that unit had been filled overnight,' Claudia said to me. People remember where they were when Prince died or Princess Diana, or when the attack on the Twin Towers happened. All of the Critical Care team remember a moment when Covid suddenly seemed real to them. For Claudia, this was that moment.

She is already getting used to the sounds of Covid Critical Care, the constant bleeps of monitors. 'In the same way as when there's a clock ticking in a room and you're used to it, you don't notice it anymore,' she said.

As mother and daughter, we are together in what is seen nationally – globally – as 'the fight against coronavirus', each of us doing our bit. Yet strangely and slowly – just like the other members of the team on the coronavirus unit – we are drawing away from anyone who is not experiencing what we are going through. We are like soldiers returning from a conflict, unable to talk about the horrors they have witnessed. We do not question it. We cannot stop to consider the effects of this daily battle.

It's tough for us, but tougher for the patients who have no visitors and are scared of this unknown and vicious virus.

21 April

Your messages and words of support continue to warm my heart, and the feedback indicates that you want to learn of the reality at the front line – although it's a war without weapons. Our doctor who worked in Afghanistan mentioned that he feels the 'dramatic level of trauma' here is somehow worse than what he experienced out there, in that war zone.

This monster is worse? This Covid war has an unseen enemy and our dwindling supply of PPE supposedly protects us. On Sunday I cared for a group of patients in a makeshift and cramped ICU on Brodie Ward: cables trailing along the ground, monitors balanced on top of ventilators, and the emergency oxygen supply for my patient was attached to the bed of another patient with rolls of green tubing that looked like a garden hose hanging off the end of the bed in this non-ICU.

The PPE is suffocating. It's hot and tight. I have a cut above my left ear from the mask's elastic. We have to shout or we cannot be heard. At one point I felt an overwhelming desire to break free and rip it all off – to lift my visor up and breathe. My nose was blocked, my throat was sore. But then an alarm went off. A patient became unstable and I was distracted.

This war requires resilience, stamina and bravery. We are operating outside our normal systems. It takes time to be a skilled professional in the Critical Care setting, and suddenly we are catapulted into this strange and new space of Covid rage.

One man died. Aged 60 and, apart from being diabetic, he was a working husband and father. A junior nurse and I held his hands as he died. We spoke to him and I tucked into his hand the photo of him at his daughter's wedding last summer. There were no curtains around his bed, no family with him. He was another Covid victim, snatched from life. The junior nurse had tears running down her face. 'This is not how it is supposed to be,' she said. I spoke to his daughter on the phone. I could hear her pain as I tried – inadequately – to describe his final moments and to reassure her that her father was not alone when he died.

He had been sedated. It is hard for the patients who are conscious, as they cannot see our faces. I hope they can see us smile at them from behind our masks. We touch their face and hands so they feel safe and we will do all we can to help them through this.

One patient I recognised and, at first, he refused to be ventilated, as he was scared. Now I am programming his ventilator, giving him medication as I look into his familiar face. Happily, he is doing well and I hope will make a full recovery.

A patient who was ventilated for 21 days left Critical Care and had been proned for much of the time (nursed while lying on his stomach to improve oxygenation). As he was wheeled out, staff lined the corridors, clapping, and he smiled, waving his arms in victory. A fantastic moment that we shared: patient and NHS staff, united in success.

There is another patient with pink gel nails, whose nail growth demonstrates the passing of time. I am sure she would be horrified to see her nails this way.

We are shattered and do what we can to ensure that we all have space to shed a private tear, or have time out to eat and drink. Hospitals always seem to be designed with only a spare inch of space. The walls are scarred from the beds and trolleys crashing into them, but the genius who designed the Atkinson Morley Wing added a large balcony. There, we can eat hot lasagne provided by CriticalNhs. It is welcome comfort food and, just for a moment, we sit on that balcony with our faces in the sun and feel like the world is normal again.

The grey, blue, green and white stainless-steel shades that we see are suddenly peppered with orange hedgehogs, purple stripes and polka-dot hair covers, sewn with love and donated by the wonderful community who support us. There is quite a fashion trend for the many nurses who look like Amish women with their hair covered by a cloth cap. The Trust tell us that these are not required as PPE. It doesn't matter: we love them and we all wear them. One of the male runners wore a pink cap with dancing kangaroos on it.

I received a text from a Portuguese nurse: 'I need some chocolate, a Coke and a new hair cover. Is there a pink one?' I was able to fulfil all three requests.

Claudia said, 'The nurses are beautiful, hilarious, tireless heroes.'

I don't know how this will end but we look forward to that day. I want to hug someone – that's what I miss.

I did have to break protocol. I found one of our young nurses in the changing room, sobbing. I cuddled her as she cried, wondering what hideous thing she had just experienced. She calmed down and I held her tight. After a few minutes she simply said, 'I miss my mum.'

Another young nurse cannot speak to her parents. 'They're scared for me and I don't want to make them more scared by telling them about the situation,' she said. 'My father is my usual support system, but now, in all of this, I can't talk to him.'

One nurse frequently stays late, after finishing her shift. Why? 'I don't want to go home. How crazy is it, not wanting to go home? But that's how I feel. And when I go home it's to eat and shower and then come back to St George's. But I just want to stay here.' We finish a shift and find reasons not to leave because going home feels wrong. At home, we feel like we are in the wrong place.

For now, this is our normal. We are adjusting and have new protocols in place and a new way of working until we have won this war.

This truly fabulous team, created after an email requesting biscuits for nurses. Their ongoing support and the support of so many friends, neighbours and far-reaching community has been phenomenal and is supporting NHS staff through this war.

*   *   *

It was a few days into Claudia's first week that a nurse said to her, 'Can you print me two wrist bands?' She printed off the wrist bands for a patient, and thought she'd take them straight to the nurse who was at a bed, behind drawn curtains. Claudia pulled back the curtains and, as she did so, she said with her usual chirpiness, 'Here are the wrist bands ...'

The nurse was washing the naked dead body of a man. 'Yeah,' she said, 'just pop them on the end of the bed.'

Claudia recoiled, shocked. Later, we talked about the incident. 'I just wasn't expecting it,' she said. 'I think if I had known ...' She felt guilty too. 'I felt as if I was witnessing a private moment. Not that he was with his family. He was being washed by one of the nurses. But it felt like a private moment that I shouldn't have seen. It wasn't really my place to see that.'

Claudia has received the brunt of relatives' anger. She answers the phones, so she is literally on the receiving end of anxious and grief-stricken family members who are forbidden from setting foot inside the hospital. One of the doctors had called a patient's family to say their loved one was dying, though not from coronavirus. Claudia was the one who listened and was kind to the woman who was shouting down the phone, 'I don't understand. You were meant to be making him better ... Because of all the Covid patients you don't care about the others that don't have it!'

Claudia, new to the job, was trying to talk this woman down, but she did not have any of the answers to her questions and there was no one to take the call because it was so chaotic and busy. The tsunami was here.

Claudia was finding it tricky on reception because, she said, 'No one ever calls to speak to the ward clerk.' Relatives of patients want to speak to a particular nurse or doctor. 'The nurse is annoyed because they're busy and the relative is annoyed because I won't give them the answers they need. But I genuinely don't have the answers to give.'

She declined a lift home, preferring to walk because, after a day of shock, she needed fresh air and some space. She had walked for about half a mile, through the near-deserted streets, and was on Tooting high street when – bang! – a car careered onto the pavement and crashed into the front of a shop. Claudia quickly phoned 999. She was asking for an ambulance to be sent when, suddenly, 20 metres down the road, a motorcycle slammed into a car. Within minutes she was at the centre of an emergency, the only witness to two incidents in an otherwise desolate corner of London.

28 April

I am a marathon runner. The sheer exhaustion I experience when running those final metres to the finish line is a similar feeling to the end of a shift on a Covid ICU, minus the exhilaration and the smile on my face – though the crowd support and the kindness of strangers is the same.

Today two total strangers connected with one another through the new and amazing community network fired up by an email from me asking for biscuits. This connection resulted in one of my lovely European nurses being lent a flat to live in for a few weeks. No rent, no bills. Just a set of keys and the Wi-Fi password. What's the catch? Absolutely none. Only the unconditional respect for Critical Care nurses.

I am astounded by the generosity and ongoing unfailing respect and gratitude for NHS staff since we left our old world and entered this new one. Thank you seems not enough for the endless stream of offers of help I receive. A 'stranger' friend said, 'You need anything, you just ask.' I did ask and he did help.

It has calmed a bit since the initial bedlam, but a level of crazy still fills the air. The Trust have put efforts into staff well-being, providing hubs to relax in that offer hot drinks and refreshments. Sadly, many of us are still too busy to pay a visit, but I definitely plan to, and there is 'real coffee'.

I miss the old way of working. The familiar spaces and machinery. I knew where the syringes were kept, where we kept the attachments for the ventilators, the property book and where we hid the keys to the cupboard.

Yesterday I didn't recognise a friend in PPE. When she spoke I couldn't hear her, as my hazmat suit covered my ears. My FFP3 mask had pushed up my glasses so I couldn't see her, and my voice was muffled through the visor so that when I spoke to her she couldn't hear me. We did laugh and bump elbows. How I took for granted our cool navy cotton scrubs and seeing our colleagues' faces.

The tide has turned somewhat. The resilience of staff has blossomed and we are settling into our new normal. We have fewer admissions and some empty beds. We are discussing our hygiene regime once we arrive home after work, bargaining with each other over various cotton scrub hats, making swaps for a particular colour or design. The mantra of 'What's for lunch?' starts from mid-morning, but none of us want to relax because the invisible monster can rear its ugly head at any moment.

I have not cried at work for years. We all take a private moment when our feelings overwhelm us or if we identify with a particular patient, but yesterday I felt a deep sadness that stayed with me all day. I cried in the office on my lunch break, worrying our lovely receptionist. I came home and cried in the shower. I then cried again. I had a large glass of wine and cried some more.

My patient was dying. As I've said before, I pride myself on my end-of-life care, but I had never imagined taping my iPhone to a drip pole with Elastoplast and angling it with a nappy towards my patient's face so that her husband and children could 'be with her' as she died. It was the best I could do, but far from good enough. The iPad intended for this use was too complicated to set up with Skype, so to connect the family as soon as possible I had to make do. Usually families stay with a patient when they die, hold their hand, lie next to them, brush their hair. This felt so wrong and crude.

This woman should not have been dying. She should have been at home nagging her children to do their homework or brush their teeth. Discussing with her husband what to have for supper. Normal Mum and family stuff.

My mood was lifted early evening when three junior nurses banged on the glass door and waved at me. 'Mama Anthea!' I could see that they were smiling beneath their masks. I am always struck by how these young women have immaculate eyeliner at the end of a shift. A passing doctor gave me a wave, too. We all look out for each other.

This pandemic is straining our health system. There are debates about PPE. Jigsaws are popular again. We clap on Thursdays, children make rainbows, neighbours chat to one another.

This is a strange time, requiring resilience, strength and hope. We can only do our best, and the staff I have the privilege of working with are doing their very best and so much more. We have many staff from Europe, India, the Philippines and from all over the world. These dedicated and fabulous people help hold up our health service.

We do have the strength to keep fighting this battle. We will go to work; you stay at home.

*   *   *

Covid has made us cry. It's an outlet for our pent-up emotions and we have been scared too that we might catch this virus. I may shed the odd tear if I identify with a particular situation, but I rarely cry. It doesn't mean I don't feel anything. Being a nurse and a mum teaches you to hold your tears back. I cry on the inside. We work in such an emotionally challenging environment that it's hardly surprising. I don't think it's ideal to cry in front of families, as it's not our grief or anxiety, but if we do need to, we find a quiet place to cry.

All of us are susceptible to our own private storm in response to the rage train we find ourselves on. Big tears and sobbing have caught most of us at some point. We are in a safe environment where support and hugs are abundant.

The last time tears rolled down my cheeks at work was shortly after I returned from maternity leave. I cared for a man who had collapsed following his mother's funeral, while having dinner with a friend. The friend called the ambulance. A CT scan revealed that he had suffered from an unrecoverable and untreatable bleed in the brain. This man lived and worked in Africa. He returned home once a year to see his mother. His mother had never met her son's wife or daughter, as she was not comfortable with the colour of her daughter-in-law's skin. His friend could not remember his wife or daughter's name and did not have an address. The patient's basic mobile phone and plane ticket were tucked safely with his passport in the side pocket of his small suitcase.

As the monitor above his bed revealed a cardiac rhythm incompatible with life, we watched him fade. His friend held his hand. He had no contactable next of kin. He was so unwell that he was not for resuscitation.

I cried, as I knew his family might be meeting his flight in Africa to welcome him home. His young daughter and her mum would be excited and standing in the arrivals hall at the airport. He died at approximately the time the flight he never boarded was due to land. Attempts by the police and Interpol to find his wife failed; with no name or address it was impossible.

This was over 20 years ago. No social media or smart-phone.

To this day, I don't know if or when his daughter and her mum ever found out what happened.

*   *   *

Claudia has settled in, even if we are in the most unsettled period of NHS history. She is carrying out duties that were not in the job description, such as finding patients' missing dentures, as well as working out why the printer will only copy in pink. She also prints the 'blood gases' – our short-hand for a sheet of paper that shows the test results of a patient's blood, such as the levels of oxygen and carbon dioxide (the gases) as well as the pH levels and acidity.

Claudia said to me one morning, 'I had this dream last night. I was sending back a parcel of clothes, and I realised

I hadn't put the receipt in the bag so wouldn't get a refund. I was chasing the postman down the road, and I got to him and said, "Please can I give you the receipt? Because otherwise they're not going to send me the money ..." And I handed him the receipt – and it was a blood gas, a really long one that was going on and on and on. I woke up and thought, *How has this infiltrated my brain?*'

She tries to keep up with answering the phones on the reception desk. They ring incessantly. She takes calls from the worried families of patients, as well as calls from theatre, the police and A&E. 'You can never let Claudia leave us,' a few of the other nurses have said to me.

It was just a question of time – a few days, in fact – before she started to see the deaths. On the reception desk there are monitors linked to nanny cameras in the cardiac operating theatres, which are now being used for coronavirus patients.

She did not want to look at the screens, which showed scenes like something out of a sci-fi movie: nurses in hazmat suits and visors tending to their sedated patients in what had been, a few weeks earlier, our windowless operating theatres. But it was hard for Claudia not to look from time to time, and at one point she sensed a flicker of movement on a screen and glanced towards it. She saw what was happening in theatre at that very moment: a patient having a cardiac arrest as doctors and nurses, clad in their unwieldy protective gear, administered *CPR, cardiopulmonary resuscitation.*

Not every patient in Critical Care is ill with coronavirus. There are still those who have suffered heart attacks, or been in serious accidents at home, at work or while travelling. So we have kept one ICU open for patients who don't have coronavirus. This is where Claudia can be found, at her desk. Though she is not at the desk all the time.

When Claudia was nine we had a girls' day out to the cinema to see *Ratatouille*, a film about a rat who aspires to become a renowned French chef. With a large bag of Maltesers, we settled down for some mother and daughter quality time.

Mid-way through the film I heard those dreaded words. 'Is there a doctor here?' a frantic, female voice called from a dark corner. I got up, telling Claudia, 'Stay there. Do not move.' I used the torch from my phone to see what was happening ... A mother had dragged her four-year-old from his seat into the aisle. She had her fingers down the child's throat. He was silent but his shoulders were jerking.

The small boy, terror in his eyes, was bleeding from his mouth and drooling pink-green slime. He'd been eating jelly sweets and inhaled one while laughing, said his mother.

I sat the boy forward, supporting his head. I wasn't sure if it was safe to perform the Heimlich manoeuvre in the dark on someone this small, so with the heel of my hand I delivered blows in an upward movement between his shoulder blades. The fourth blow dislodged the wedged jelly frog that was obstructing his airway, along with more slime and his recently consumed lunch which projected over my knees. He spluttered and screamed – a wonderful sound to hear after the silence of choking.

I washed my hands and knees, although Claudia and I finished the film to a faint odour of vomit. Poor Claudia. She was totally traumatised and has never again watched *Ratatouille*.

MAY 2020

5 May

This weekend I spent some time gardening, with my son Peter at the piano belting out 'Viva la Vida' by Coldplay. It's great to be home, as I am exhausted to the core.

On Monday Claudia and I did the *Good Morning Britain* interview. It was slightly surreal sitting on the sofa at home and staring at a blank screen, my laptop balanced on books on top of a storm lantern on our coffee table, and with a shaky connection that meant we frequently only heard half the questions from a faceless voice. 'Keep looking at the laptop camera' was the only instruction from a *GMB* producer.

I remain overwhelmed by the generosity my colleagues and I have received, and it just keeps on. People ask, 'How are you?' This is an impossible question to answer, as there is no explanation for what we are doing. I just know this: Critical Care nurses are truly incredible warriors.

We have relocated one of the temporary Covid areas to a cardiac ward with more space and a better layout, to be morphed into yet another Critical Care unit. Manoeuvring and transporting one critically ill patient in a lift with ventilators, pumps, monitors and other emergency equipment, often bleeping and buzzing, can be challenging at the best of times, and the lifts are only a few centimetres wider than the beds, the over-sensitive automated doors opening and closing while drip poles and the patient's cot sides and other paraphernalia become jammed. The lift alarm screams, while brute force is required to propel the bed forward over the lift threshold, which is never exactly the same level as the floor you have alighted from.

All done, we then eat delicious homemade raspberry and lemon cake, courtesy of The Jam Tarts.

I remember giggling when I was pregnant, having to wedge my bump into the small space sideways when my patient required a CT scan. The nurses effortlessly moved 14 patients to the floor below without fuss, as they are competent and trained to do so. They were then rewarded with beautiful cupcakes.

The following day several fantastic support nurses and Health Care Assistants (HCAs) organised, cleared and deep cleaned an eerily empty space that had seen much mayhem, severe illness and death over the past weeks, when the Covid-19 tsunami sent its first wave. An abandoned pair of goggles lay on the floor next to a square of gauze: the remnants of what had been.

Now the 30-bed ward is empty and abandoned. It is still and it echoes. I stood and took in the impossible silence. In all my career I had never seen a ward devoid of patients, noise and clutter. The alarms of monitors, ventilators and pumps no longer sounded their demands, and I shed a tear as I remembered the ordered war zone and what this space had witnessed and absorbed.

There is a pause while we prepare for the next surge as people break their lockdown. We still have many critically ill patients and take Covid patients from other hospitals who are retrieved by our newly established critical care retrieval service and amazing outreach team. Empty beds are prepared, ventilators are calibrated and fresh linen awaits its next victim who may today be chatting with family at home, running on the common, or at work – perhaps a key worker – unaware that they are next.

We have patients a moment away from death, and never lose faith that some will recover. Machinery, drugs and expertise are willing them on. Some patients, now improving, are delirious and try to climb out of bed, their circadian rhythm upended. Managing these patients is challenging and communication is tricky in full PPE. A combination of chemical restraint, nurse power and kindness keeps them safe.

One patient said he was late for work and needed to go. He kept trying to climb out of bed, pulling at the drips and cables attached to him. Another man FaceTimed his wife to say he was feeling better and added, 'The lockdown has done you no favours, my dear. You have gained weight.'

His wife laughed and replied, 'It's true. I have.'

We keep crying. One of the doctors admitted he had gone home and sobbed. A senior staff nurse told me, 'After my night shifts I sit in my car and cry.' Another said, 'I work scared.' I told one of the nurses I had cried. 'You, Mama?' she replied, shocked that this wild beast had affected me too. 'I come by and give you an Italian squeeze.' And she did.

I salute our nurses, who show kindness, resilience and compassion. Our entire team. The doctors who work unrelenting hours under immense pressure, the ward clerk who returns a found phone to a patient. The porters and runners who distribute our food, the matrons who coordinate in the background and all frontline workers and my many 'stranger friends'.

One of Australia's most successful rock bands, Birds of Tokyo, in collaboration with the West Australian Symphony Orchestra, performed 'Unbreakable' for frontline workers. And we are unbreakable. From Earlsfield to Australia, we are supported, and Critical Care nurses are the new heroes.

> *'No one can make you change who you are,*
> *No one can take one beat from your heart,*
> *When you're standing tall*
> *You're unbreakable.'*

12 May

Mayhem and trauma have abated. We have enough Critical Care staff. We have enough support staff who have been 'upskilled' to work alongside trained ICU nurses. We have devised a system and a new routine. It's not ideal and it's not sustainable in our 'red zone that soon became the blue zone'.

(Red zone was the area for Covid patients, green for non-Covid, and amber for those not confirmed but not suspected; they then changed the red to blue and added in yellow – all very confusing. Currently a blue area is an area of ICU that is for Covid-positive patients.)

I cared for a man whose son said to me on the phone, 'I am not worried about dignity. You must keep him going until his last breath.' We are all dislocated. This son has no idea of what happens behind the walls of a Critical Care unit. His seemingly uncaring comment only demonstrates that he doesn't know how it is on any level. He has no idea that his father has had his life taken already. Machinery makes his lungs inspire and expire. He is not breathing anymore. Drugs make his heart beat. A filtration machine works on behalf of his kidneys. Another machine cools his blood. His blood chemistry is not compatible with life. He is suspended between now and death, and he will die with strangers. Strong, kind, fabulous strangers.

I feel as if I am in a spaceship. A Covid bubble. We wave through the glass window at our allocated runner for the day if we need something, and moments after they have gone to retrieve the unpronounceable item, you remember something else you need.

Death is the toughest thing. We have become adept at using a variety of items to secure iPads in place for FaceTime calls. Some families play music, pray or chant. A 12-year-old played her dad the latest piece she had learned on the piano, and told him that she had been practising her scales without Mummy nagging.

We took a transfer from an out-of-area hospital, and in a bag was a photo of the patient looking healthy and happy on a beach with his wife. These reminders of normality give me a pain in my heart.

The PPE is too much now. Our chins are red, our noses sore. I find the visor, mask and scrub hat are all tight, hot and irritating after a while. Snot runs down your face. One pregnant nurse vomited into her mask. The coloured scrub hats are as popular as ever and nurses have developed different ways of tying them up. The Amish look has become that of a 1940s housewife or Second World War land girl – or a baker or chef. The Italian nurses seem to pull this look off quite well, with bright colours, large bows and immaculate eye make-up.

Your support continues. On the seventy-fifth anniversary of VE Day – last Friday – an opera singer sang his heart out from the back of a truck that pulled up outside the Covid ICU and wards. Cupcakes were handed out. Staff and patients stood on the balcony and nurses waved from the windows. Even an ambulance leaving the hospital paused for the sound of Vera Lynn's 'We'll Meet Again' – somehow so apt.

We still cry. One of our consultants cried. A junior doctor redeployed from another area was astonished to see an ex-military male senior doctor blubbering in the office and had no idea how to respond. He reversed out of the room quickly.

We didn't sign up for this. From cleaners to consultants, we all have a different perspective. One senior nurse said, 'Being in charge is like flying a fighter jet in combat.'

I spoke to a patient who had been so sick and intubated six times. I honestly didn't expect him to survive. Heart warmed by his incredible progress as he sat on the edge of the bed, supported by the physiotherapists, I told him he looked amazing. He said, 'You think? I can't even hold up my fucking head ...' Later, I made him tea. He couldn't drink it but I dipped a mouth swab in it. 'Not Earl Grey,' he said.

A woman brought cake for the Critical Care nurses. She had not seen her husband since an ambulance took him to hospital on 2 April. No visitors are permitted but, as his bed was by the window, she stood outside and we held up his hand so that she could see him wave.

We now wait to see what happens next. Be alert! Brace yourself. We may need to board the rollercoaster again.

International Nurses Day – respect and thank you to our nurses from all over the world. We actually couldn't do it without you.

One of the young nurses has taken up painting by numbers. 'Usually,' she says, 'I am the least creative person in the entire world.' But now she is painting on her days off. 'I have to get my mind off it,' she explains. She lives with three other girls. Or rather, she lived with three other girls. They work in PR, and when Covid came they thought, We're living with a nurse who works in ICU. We're going to die. They packed their bags and went home to their parents. So now she lives alone.

18 May

The best rendition of the Mad Hatter's tea party was when we yet again relocated 16 patients so that another one of our ICUs could be deep cleaned.

Seeing long-term patients improving and leaving the ward after a precarious and stormy Covid journey is always heart-warming, but there was not a dry eye in the house when a patient left Critical Care for the ward after a full recovery. A man we thought would die despite our best care, he was wheeled out to a standing ovation, from ward clerk to consultant. He high-fived as he passed. It was magical.

Our new normal has settled; we are adapting to our non-ICU. The 'can do' staff have devised new ways. A vomit bowl has been converted into an iPad stand (since writing this, we now have a fabulous gadget to hold them in place). Beds are manoeuvred to create the space we need to house all the machinery required. The Weetabix stash has been relocated and ventilation tubing and filters are in their place in perfectly labelled boxes. Nurses are ingenious and practical.

Despite Covid-19, Critical Care still admits regular patients into our green zone: a teenager who drank too much at a party (despite lockdown); an elderly woman hit by a car; a brain haemorrhage in a young man. Patients with a burst appendix, an overdose, asthma attack, a cardiac arrest, stroke, motorbike accident, a fall downstairs or off a roof. The many individuals who arrive at our door to be fixed and cared for, who recover or don't. St George's is still open for business and these patients can be cared for in a safe Covid-free space.

Since the war began, our head of nursing and matrons have stayed all night on occasion to plan and ensure we have supplies and safe staffing levels. Doctors who do not work in Critical Care have learned new skills. Cleaners have to don full PPE to empty a bin or clean the floor, as do the porters who transfer people, equipment, documents and bodies to their next destination. NHS staff are superheroes fuelled by the compassion and support (and cake) from all of you.

One Spanish nurse finished her 12-hour night shift, removed her PPE, her face lined from the mask but with red lipstick intact, which matched her scrub hat. 'But of course,' she shrugged when I commented.

We have to try to find hope, somewhere in this mess. This is a collective endeavour beyond sweat and exhaustion by NHS staff who are coping because they have to. Terrifying for everyone, for the entire world. Staff who had no idea this pandemic would become their way of life. This contagion has brought out our essential humanity, but we did not prepare for and could not have predicted it. We are living day by day. We link like an orchestra, connecting together as a symphony to provide the best possible patient care.

At the start, back in March when the floodgates opened, there were criteria set for who should be admitted, who should be palliated. We had to ensure there were beds for those who needed them. We have space now.

I recall a conversation with a woman who had a poor medical history and tested positive for Covid-19. The consultant asked in the kindest way, did she want to be ventilated? Did she want CPR? What level of medical intervention was acceptable to her? It's a tough conversation to have but so much better to talk with the patient directly so that, should they deteriorate, we know what they have chosen.

The woman wanted to discuss this with her sister, and to know that she would never be in pain. And she asked that her niece take care of her cat. A DNR order was instituted and discarded once she improved and was discharged to the ward.

Covid patients surrender themselves to us. It isn't just Covid-19 that attacks them. Perhaps a cytokine storm overwhelms them, a bacterial pneumonia, a bleed on the brain or, mostly, multi-organ failure.

The nurses are there for them. We move a bed next to a window so the patient can see the trees. A patient with learning difficulties watches *Mr Tumble* on a loop. Mouth swabs are dipped in orange juice. A senior sister on night shifts always gives a foot massage to a particular patient to help him sleep. It is calmer and quieter, but the cracks are beginning to show.

'My head spins, my heart pounds in my chest and I can't breathe.'

'I have nightmares every night.'

These nurses are now receiving counselling but the senior staff are alert for others that need support. We care for each other, laugh together, cry together, and there is nothing like a full-on PPE hug. Hugs are a basic human need. I miss hugging my non-work friends and family. Nurses are lucky. We get more hugs than anyone from someone who totally *gets it*.

Don't forget us. This has not gone. If the predicted surge doesn't happen we are very, very lucky. But if it does happen then we know how it feels to drown. This time we have a few life jackets.

For now, we focus on recovery and rehabilitation for some patients or enable a good death for those who will not survive.

I hear my emails are spreading far and wide, and people ask if there is anything they can do to help. There is. I challenge you all at this time with these three things to help us and help you.

1. Talk to your family about your end-of-life wishes.
2. Talk to your family about organ donation.
3. Always wear a helmet on a bike. If you are on a family cycle in a park and one of you cycles downhill fast and your chain snaps and you hit the ground headfirst, at speed, a helmet may just make the difference. No helmet and there may be one less person in your family.

30 May

There are not enough Critical Care nurses. We have so many nurses from other areas who have stepped up and are stretching themselves way beyond their comfort zone. Senior staff have had to adapt to a different way. A dental nurse, a dementia specialist nurse, a nurse from theatre or endoscopy – competent in their own area but suddenly removed from their context – they are having to learn on the hoof, and my shattered team need to direct, guide and supervise them. Mostly we embrace this, but it's exhausting for us all.

I take charge and search the PPE-masked faces to spot my own familiar staff. Yesterday the result of displaced staff had disastrous consequences.

For those of us in charge, there is an internal monologue in our heads – we have to keep a grip on admissions, transfers, discharges, deaths. Staffing levels, drug supplies, equipment needed and changes and requirements in each individual patient's plan of care. Ventilator alterations and haemofiltration exchange adjustments. Weaning plans, rehabilitation plans, trips to MRI. Who needs proning or deproning, and who is unstable and who is going to die? We need to know who the staff are and what knowledge and skills they have or don't have. Staffing for the next shift needs to be confirmed and sickness or absence recorded. We balance our ICU staff, distributing them as best we can. We communicate with staff, family and the entire team involved in the care of each patient. Microbiology, haematology, blood bank, pharmacy, ward clerk, CT scan, X-ray, technicians, porters. All the people and departments involved in a person's care. It is exhausting and our brains spin.

Who do we run for first? A patient who is desaturating? Another one who is waking up because the sedation is wearing off? Another one whose blood pressure is dropping?

I am sleeping so badly, we all are. Braced for the next punch. I have learned so much about the aetiology of Covid-19, its progress and supportive treatment. Having seen a multitude of different reasons for admission to Critical Care over the years, we are fast learning about a new disease process unfamiliar to us. In that respect this is easier. All the patients have the same issue, similar symptoms, similar care and treatment. Unrelenting. There's less madness, but the patients are still arriving and there are patients who have been with us for weeks, but we are coping.

After 40 days on ICU, a patient left last week. For many of those 40 days he was ventilated and proned. 'No clapping,' he said. It was all too overwhelming. 'Covid didn't get me. I got Covid.' We have this pinned up on the wall in the red zone. We all have 'battle fatigue'. The space to think is now available and we are beginning to unravel.

Sadly, I have been a victim of the 'crying thing' again. It's actually a relief to cry. I was in a safe space with my family, and my son – unprompted – gave me a kiss (this never normally happens).

I heard that on one of our Covid areas, in order to prone a patient to save her life, she required an emergency caesarian to deliver her premature baby. Covid seems to badly affect some pregnant women, presumably because their immunity is lower. Her tiny baby was too early to survive.

I am not sure if we will have a surge like the first wave that hit, but this virus keeps revealing its victims. Patients who cannot speak English must be so scared. We rely on a member of staff speaking the same language. One woman was on holiday in London when Covid struck her. It will be a long time before she returns to her home in Poland.

Our world feels broken. There is an economic downturn. Shops are boarded up. I cycled through central London last week and saw how it is now owned by runners, cyclists and walkers. The streets are quiet but the parks are crowded, as if there is a festival on.

Behind the doors of St George's we plan and devise new protocols, and every week this changes. We have adapted. We navigate the obstacles, we continue on, mustering up fresh energy and perspective. Frequently moving patients, opening new areas, disrupting staff. Clean areas, dirty areas, Covid zones.

The highlight of the ninth clap was a trip to the helipad at St George's. We clapped for frontline workers, and the BBC filmed us. It was an amazing experience to share with Claudia.

We remain challenged by a different space at work. Nurses are resilient, as a senior consultant pointed out, and we don't complain about the work. We complain about the lack of parking and office space.

For now things have improved but we wait and see. I am emotionally robust but this has hit me hard. The NHS is usually stretched to the limit but now has to cope with the arrival of patients who have been 'hanging in there' at home. They are really unwell and it's not always possible to fix them. They are reluctant and scared to come to hospital to be treated, and there is no cure.

Please remember, as your world starts returning to some semblance of normal, that it's not over. Please keep washing your hands. Behind the orange brick walls, we are still fighting this. Our incredible, unbreakable and fabulous team shine brightly.

JUNE 2020

4 June

A few weeks ago the discount at the local butcher was 20 per cent. I was smiled at when I skipped the queue at the supermarket. I felt emotionally warmed by the Thursday clap, especially when leaving the hospital after a day at work. Ambulances would flash their lights and sound their sirens; staff and patients and local residents would cheer.

Not now. Now 20 per cent is 10 per cent. I get glared at when I produce my NHS ID at the shop entrance, as the queue for the next person in line has now become one person longer. People have stopped clapping, which had already slowed, as 8 p.m. could interrupt the evening meal, bath time or a Zoom call with friends. Nurses now hate the clap. The novelty has worn off – it means nothing now. Lockdown is seemingly lifted. People are distracted by the need for a holiday or haircut; they're fed up and ready to get back to their abandoned lives.

NHS staff now spring to mind when we are needed. When you want a doctor or end up in A&E with a persistent cough and difficulty breathing, or another minor or serious illness or accident.

But that is OK. Perhaps we should move on and get back to normal. We are appreciated by the majority of people who, in fact, are our patients – past, present and future.

Inside the Covid bubble at work the PPE is plentiful. There is a system in place. The NHS love to have a process. Staff know where their new workplace is. We are organised. Shelves are labelled and cupboards tidy. The Covid ICUs run parallel to the regular ICU that cares for the usual flow of non-Covid patients. Elective surgery has restarted and the small steps of recovery are beginning to emerge.

We have liaison nurses allocated to update families, but now I telephone the family myself to directly update them or pass on a message. I have time and can learn about the patient I have been caring for. It's lovely to pass on the message that the garden at home is looking great, the roses are out, or Sarah has had a baby boy. Recovering patients without visitors need the minute detail of home. They are often too tired for a FaceTime call.

Mentally, we are not the same as we were at the beginning of this fight. Our bond is stronger. The level of teamwork is incredible and we have gone slightly off-piste with some pre-existing policies that are no longer relevant, devised before the madness or created by someone disconnected from the truth. We swerve the red tape and have devised practical solutions to some of the obstacles Covid presented us with.

A bottle of Champagne cracked open with close senior colleagues in a back garden in the sun was the absolute best therapy – letting rip with friends who understand. To be in charge, to lead the day to day is tough. I am supporting junior staff, supporting strangers who are 'picking it up' as they go along.

I am used to working with a skilled, knowledgeable, experienced medical team, or teaching and mentoring a junior team within a purpose-built environment. I am not used to working with staff unqualified in the Critical Care speciality. I am grateful for them, but at the same time shocked, worried and frustrated because learning on the hoof in such an area is far from ideal. There is skilled witchery involved in optimising a person's blood gases by fine-tuning their ventilator settings.

There is a glorious madness to our days. Getting caught up in a gown which is tricky to don in a hurry. My waist tie is always in a knot. Masks tangled in hair, glasses and visors. Clanging heads with a colleague as we temporarily underestimate the visor space between us. Having a conversation with a stranger who turns out to be one of your favourite people once the mask is off. Mishearing, 'Do you want to go for a coffee?' as, 'Do you know where the mop is?'

Nurses are loving, physical people and we work in such close proximity in sometimes intimate and emotionally challenging situations. We hug each other a lot and I am seeing nurses kiss each other. How lucky I am to have so many hugs and a closeness to my colleagues, many of whom are my friends.

A Covid patient is admitted to hospital. He is an intravenous drug user who also smokes crack cocaine. He is recovering and will be discharged to the ward soon. I asked, 'Will you get back on the stuff again?'

He answered, 'Nah! That's a mug's game. I am done with all that. I think you could say I've been given a second chance. Bloody good thing I got this Covid bug.'

Covid bug?! Fantastic that the enormity of Covid has had such a positive life-changing impact on his frail, war-torn body.

It's true that this affects the black and ethnic minority groups of people, and those who have a high BMI or hypertension (elevated blood pressure) or diabetes. However, they are definitely not the only ones. Last week we had a young mum who had just had a baby. A colleague who works at another hospital cared for a young, fit marathon runner who sadly died. I have seen, or directly nursed, previously fit and healthy people of all ages. A scientist, an actor, a musician, a bus driver, a nurse, a chef, a father, a gardener, a domestic, a research scientist, a lawyer, a teacher, a secretary and a member of staff from *Topshop*. Anyone can be affected, just regular people. Anyone can die.

Those admitted to ICU for organ support may be mended by our brilliance and newly acquired Covid knowledge. In fact, we are seeing more and more people survive. We are getting better and better at this. We now know what Covid does to a person's body and how we can support and treat their symptoms.

It is better but it continues to be here. We are still admitting Covid patients. In March, when I did a 14-hour day (should have been 12 hours; I was paid for 11.5 hours), when two out of my six patients died, when my phone was strapped to a drip pole, when my support nurse kept crying, when my ears were ringing as I felt so dehydrated, my bladder full and my heart heavy … Well, that has all abated. But, still bruised from an experience I thought was not possible, my concern for my colleagues, our frustration at the lack of many things – that remains.

I started writing this back in March to thank you, then to inform you, and now, in some strange way, it helps me to write it. My writing has become cathartic. It is a way for me to relive the thoughts and feelings in my head.

Thank you endlessly for your support. To my friends who tolerate my silence, understand my need to complain or cry or say nothing, but deliver a treat or message regularly without receiving a reply. The waves and kisses blown by friends I pass while on a run. Usually a positive person, I sometimes feel angry but am not sure why – often minor issues trigger it. This week I felt mightily annoyed that a qualified Critical Care nurse I have worked with for 15 years had the wrong size scrubs because a 'helper' had been given the last pair in her size. I need to be calm, take a breath. One day this will be over.

We are prepared for a surge if one happens, and quietly and tentatively we are trying to get the hospital back to some sort of normality. Freshly deep cleaned, stocked and waiting to go.

This week Claudia spent time looking for an elderly man's property, retracing his journey around the Critical Care areas. He was low in mood and missing his wife. Claudia eventually found it, and he was thrilled to be reunited with his long-lost dentures and electric shaver, more so than his phone and wallet, which were also found. Such joy on his face.

Last Wednesday three nurses spent two hours combing, detangling and de-matting the acquired dreadlocks from a woman who had spent weeks being bed-bound, her thick locks coated with sweat, blood, dead skin, sticky medication, milky feed, vomit and saliva. Washed, conditioned and tangle free, her luxurious hair shone. Nurses are superstars in their own quiet and unseen way.

13 June

My last email seemed to provoke a particularly huge response for some reason. I am not some magnificent human. I am just an experienced and senior nurse giving you a glimpse of what happens within the walls of Critical Care units within one of the UK's largest hospitals.

Don't put me on a pedestal, because when this is over and we all go back to normal I am just a regular person: a neighbour, friend, relative, local mum, and just one of a huge group of individuals who found themselves unexpectedly on the front line. No choice. I am told, actually, that I can be very annoying. One of my closest friends tells me I am weird. And everyone tells me I talk loudly!

Our postman visibly stepped back when he saw me today. One of our nurses has had her toddler banned from nursery because she is a frontline worker. Other parents feel uncomfortable that their children will mix with her child. Not one of our own Critical Care nurses ended up as a Covid patient in our department, and most of us tested antibody negative. Our infection control procedures and PPE are robust.

We are not really superheroes and there is no nurse emoji on your phone. (Ha! There is now – added since Covid.)

One of our patients who just skirted death is regretting his lifelong smoking habit. He has been on intensive care for 50 days and, weaned from the ventilator, he has started to eat. One of our nurses hotfooted it to the corner shop and bought him a Magnum, as he really fancied some ice cream. In fact, four of our long-term recovering patients ate ice cream on Friday. Looking at their faces made all that's happened OK for a moment.

At the peak of the pandemic – when we were two Critical Care nurses to six patients (it's usually 1:1), with an endoscopy and dental nurse helping, a willing runner outside the room collecting what we needed – two patients died, one patient had a cardiac arrest, we proned another patient and one had an emergency tracheostomy. I needed six arms, as a young man was delirious and trying to climb out of bed. It is hard even to remember, as it makes me feel anxious. A surreal memory of something extreme, impossible – and it still haunts us.

Now we wait to see how and if this revs up again. Any more Covid casualties? We expect a resurgence and take Covid patients from smaller hospitals, but so far it is quiet; we have empty beds and we wait. On Tuesday there were no Covid admissions to the hospital. The recent protests, crowded parks and packed beaches cause us concern, but we just have to wait and see.

Day to day, the plan changes. Green unit, amber unit, red unit. The traffic lights are irritating. The systems are slow, the internet cuts out and there are many meetings. Staff are moved around like counters on a board game. There are layers of management and senior individuals who make decisions. Some are not in the building but working from home as per the government's instruction; non-clinical staff in East Grinstead or New Malden. How can they have any real idea of what is happening on the shop floor? No one can. If you can't see it, you can't possibly know, and, once seen, you cannot unsee it.

We need it to surge or return to normal, but somehow I don't think Critical Care will ever be normal again. I miss those days.

I popped up to the ward to visit two patients discharged from the red zone. They both cried. After weeks on Critical Care they feel homesick for the masked faces they trust. We invested in these patients and gave them a part of ourselves, and it was not just for their benefit that I went to see them.

Nursing is in my blood. When I was about seven years old I would sit on our front porch and wait for my mother to return from her night shift in A&E. I loved the stories. I knew I would be a nurse. It wasn't really a decision; it's like falling in love – you can't help yourself. Now I am the one telling the stories. Some nurses fall out of love, but I never did.

* * *

Viruses change over time, sometimes in significant ways. Scientists are working on vaccines and there is hope. The most prudent path is to be prepared. We recognise Covid symptoms now and medics carefully examine chest X-rays for the Covid clues – the ground-glass patterned areas in the lungs. Currently we have very few Covid-positive level 3 patients (complex patients who require advanced multi-organ support).

Covid areas wait, and the other areas have recommenced elective surgery, while normal Critical Care services have resumed. When I see Claudia she is always doing something extraordinary. Yesterday she witnessed the signing of a will for a patient. Claudia said, 'She wasn't concerned about dying but just wanted to get things in order.' Claudia said it was the strangest moment – to stand in a cubicle with a Roman Catholic priest, both of them wearing scrubs and PPE, while witnessing the last will and testament of a dying patient.

Claudia has been incredible. I am so proud of my daughter. She remains the IT genius. A PC wouldn't work in the green zone and my matron asked her to take a look – she simply switched it on! Critical Care nurses operate the most complex machinery and calculate drug doses at nanograms per kilogram per minute, titrating drugs to gain a precise blood pressure or blood-glucose level. But when it comes to simple IT solutions, we're terrible.

Nurses and doctors are copers. Many of us are trying to heal. In some ways it's worse. Before, we just got on with it:

no choice, no time to think. But now this fantastic team have time to unravel. We seem fine, but scratch the surface and we are not really. We have built incredible bonds and I am in awe of our Critical Care consultant team, who have been strong, directed patient care, and have at all times, like never before, supported the nurses, whom they recognise are the ones that care for the patients.

Our European nurses are booking trips home. When I left for home last night there were only seven patients left in our red zone. Cardiac surgery has resumed, neuro patients are on the neuro unit. We are beginning to allow visitors to see patients at the end of their life ... and Pret is fleecing us again.

Perhaps we are nearing the end. Or perhaps not.

21 June

I love to run. I ran a half-marathon shortly before Covid took over my life and I am just back to running longer distances. Running clears my mind and it feels great to escape. It is my therapy and my time alone to recalibrate.

I am concerned for our mental health – anxiety, fear, exhaustion and insomnia. Everyone seems fine, but we all feel the same. We are not OK at all. I have taken numerous calls from broken nurses who need sympathy, support and grati- tude. A friend called me after having a panic attack. Fine at work, but once home felt 'displaced and scared'. We are offered free counselling and many staff have seen one of our lovely counsel team members, but it's hard to describe the war we have experienced without speaking our medical language, and how do we explain? One nurse told me she 'plays it down' during these sessions, as our memories are too brutal to share. Our nurses don't tell their family the truth in case they worry.

My nephew told me, 'I don't read your emails because they are too hard to read.'

I said, 'Actually, it's too hard to do.'

Patient-wise, it's better: seemingly no surge yet. Our Covid areas only have a few patients remaining; they have been with us so long they have tested Covid-negative. Yesterday my area – General ICU – looked almost back to normal: police guarding a patient under arrest; patients going to and returning from theatre; physiotherapists helping a patient walk, promoting an improvement in function, rehabilitation and independence; non-Covid, regular patients being cared for by our own magnificent Critical Care team.

Discarded blue gloves and disposable masks now litter the streets. Healthcare professionals find this absurd, as these flimsy masks will not protect us; they will damage the environment, litter the streets and give a false sense of security. I imagine them getting dropped onto the floor on trains or toilets and then worn against a person's face or kept in a pocket, warm and moist with crumbs and saliva – attracting what they are supposed to repel.

Staff are required to complete a complex risk-assessment form. We already risked our lives, without any choice – it's a bit late now!

We have spent enough time in PPE that I feel disinclined to wear a mask on the street. I saw someone in Tooting lift his mask with a gloved hand to spit on the ground. He then scratched his ear and replaced his mask.

Support bubbles, barbecues and social groups are unlocking people's lives. There are glimpses of normal all around, and it feels good. One nurse had a beer outside a pub. She sent me a message: 'It felt so, so nice.'

We are the coronavirus heroes. I have never been particularly militant, but I hear we will receive a medal from the government. That's nothing. We need more, so much more. Even a significant pay rise would not help entirely. We have been smashed. I am strong, robust and laugh a lot, but I will never be the same again. I will always carry a part of this with me, as will our many superb people, from our clinical director for Critical Care to our cleaners. We all played a part.

The Trust leads with social distancing and 'please wear a mask when entering the hospital' signs. Front-desk staff yell at anyone entering the building without a mask gagging them. Regular communication bulletins are sent out to inform staff of updated policy. The Trust is endlessly trying to keep up with government and health-and-safety guidelines, emotionally distanced and naive about how it really is for those in direct contact. The clinical staff, while on the edge themselves, are in the privileged position because they totally 'get it'. We are touching the patient. How can anyone else possibly know or fully understand?

Social distancing cannot apply in such a space. The contact with patients and each other is incredible, and being at work with those who have shared so much is like being with family.

Pecan slices, homemade cakes and biscuits and those sausage rolls are lovely treats that keep appearing, and the Trust continue to supply crisps, bottled water, biscuits and sandwiches. A toasted-sandwich maker makes these sandwiches delicious, and a Nespresso machine donated by a friend made many nurses smile. I notice the oat and coconut milks in the fridge, brought in by the nurses to add to their coffee.

I try to spend time chatting, to express our appreciation to whichever lovely person drops off a delivery of treats. The fantastic team of temporary ward clerks help me carry them, after waiting patiently (many of them university students, including Claudia).

I apologised the other day for keeping them waiting prior to their efficient delivery of sweet treats to our Critical Care areas. One of them said, 'Don't worry. It reminds me of waiting for my mum after church.' He made me laugh so much.

We continue, surge or no surge. Surgery is backed up, and those who avoided coming to hospital and have deteriorated at home now need us. It's always busy, always fast paced, always excellent and frequently hilarious. Critical Care delivered by the most awesome gold-standard team.

It's all OK and it's not OK at all.

Today a patient said, 'I was in a restaurant in March having lunch with my mum after a long ride on my horse. I had a cough and felt tired. Now it is June. What happened to me?'

Thank you to my community and ever-expanding circle for being there for us and for not stopping – just yet.

28 June

The best part of Covid is the strong bonds we form, and no amount of tutting from a non-clinical member of staff when we are seen in our Critical Care space hugging our colleagues can make me step back a couple of metres.

It's a risk-versus-benefit thing. Who knew that hugs were needed for survival? But they are. They have supported us through the death of our patients, the wretchedness we feel, the isolation and exhaustion. We are brave and strong and emotional and pay no attention to social distancing, as we have all been wallowing in the same petri dish for months.

I connected a ventilated and awake patient to the haemo-filtration machine. I needed forceps to unscrew the caps that were attached tightly to the catheter in her neck. My lovely patient held the clamps and passed them back and forth to me as I needed them – my invaluable assistant supporting her own care. The bond we develop with our patients is outstand-ing. Critical Care patient turnover is usually fairly fast, but the Covid patients are with us for weeks on end and we get to know them so well.

A Tamil-speaking doctor translated for a 60-day resident on Covid ICU. The patient was low in mood and we were finally able to learn from the Tamil translation that 'hospital food tastes like shit!' A quick call to the patient's sister remedied the situation. A few hours later she dropped off the homemade chickpea curry and rice cake he longed for.

Last weekend I felt close to tears the entire day. In order to permanently double our Critical Care capacity we need to recruit more staff. I run the nurse recruitment and care for patients and take charge, and I just felt overwhelmed while trying to swerve the ever-emerging PTSD.

Nurses' resilience, persistence and, at the same time, gentleness have been an example to humankind. Staff are starting to plan trips home and I have set interviews for promotion before they go, in the hope that they will return. We invest time and finances into educating and training Critical Care nurses. NHS England say we must increase our footprint – our Critical Care beds – to serve London better. But the meetings and planning and meetings go on, and nothing is decided or agreed or signed off in these Microsoft Teams meetings by all the people working from home: finance, operational leaders and directors of this, that and the other; those who decide how we should run our hospital, which, despite everything, runs itself thanks to the medical staff.

On Tuesday evening I was blindsided by love. My junior team arranged a surprise and showered me with gifts, cards, claps and thank yous for being their Mama Anthea. I was (for once) speechless, overwhelmed by the very best hand-picked by me – a team of total superstars.

One of our senior nurses – my colleague and friend who has been an inspiration and support, leading and educating – left her last shift on Covid ICU to clapping and cheering by staff who lined the corridors, the same as we did for our patients when they left our Covid unit having survived. We all cried. Clapping has a whole new meaning for me now.

I have been wondering if I should stop my emails soon or wean them as we weaned our patients from their ventilators.

On 26 June 2020 the last patient left Covid Critical Care. Our red zone is now empty. Abandoned. After three months and one day, not one Covid patient requires ICU care. Spaces were cleaned and equipment returned, and our incredible team, created overnight four months ago, ate pizza together, reminiscing. I almost felt sad, but it was tinged with relief – this time had ended. Our WhatsApp group brimmed with comments of camaraderie. We were catapulted back to our regular place of work, and our temporary support staff were discarded. So weird, so strange. Our new normal now gone.

One of our support workers said when she started working on Critical Care that she had boarded the Covid Express train. The train has arrived at its destination now. We treated so many patients on Critical Care and lost so many. But count-less patients survived – some against all odds, and many of those have now gone home. Some will suffer from Long Covid and some will be left with long-term health issues, but many will live their regular lives, and their stay at St George's will fade to become a distant memory.

Will the Covid Express run again? Is the enemy hiding behind the wall, ready to fire again?

We wait.

We are invincible.

JULY 2020

4 July

Email number 15? My life changed 15 emails ago, 15 weeks ago.

Well, it was the last email last week, but the reaction I received was incredible, so perhaps I should keep going for a bit.

I interviewed our junior band 5 staff nurses for promotion this week: 34 junior nurses who deserve the promotion, who have given their all and so much more through this terrifying ordeal. One nurse returned from maternity leave after ten months off, breast-feeding and catapulted into the Covid rage. Every time she went home she was scared she would infect her baby. She didn't.

One of the interview questions I asked was, 'Name one positive outcome you experienced as a Critical Care nurse during Covid-19?'

Thirty-four nurses who have been tried and tested and pushed beyond their limit. They each mentioned teamwork, friendship, bonds, resilience. 'We are like family,' said one of them.

On Wednesday I am back on my usual day in my usual area – General ICU. Already it looks totally back to normal, apart from the colourful scrub hats nurses continue to wear. FFP3 masks are replaced with regular masks, which cause my glasses to steam up because the fit is not as robust as the FFP3 masks.

The unit is noisy with alarms and chatter. A patient is nursed on a mattress on the floor to protect him after his two-day binge on spice (synthetic cannabis). Trauma patients from motorbike accidents occupy several beds, and there is a patient in following cancer surgery, an overdose, an elderly woman dying. Back to normal. Our wrung out and not-quite-healed nurses are caring in their usual majestic way – though there is a dearth of European nurses, as many have gone home to family for a few weeks.

Our Covid escalation area will resume normal activity on Monday as a cardiac ward. Hours were spent clearing it of equipment and Critical Care kit, and then it was deep cleaned until spotless. I couldn't even enter the empty space yesterday, as it was our war zone. It's eerie and strange, and the calm and quiet of freshly made beds and no clutter is so different from before. But for many of us the atmosphere and the dust from what happened is impregnated into the walls.

My last day on Ben Weir Ward, the second make-do ICU. I took the clock off the wall, as a friend had bought it for me. I picked up my visor (bought on Amazon as the ones we had were too big) and left. We saw so much through those visors.

We feel naked without PPE. We depended on it, then we tolerated it, and now, bizarrely, we miss it. A plastic apron seems so flimsy.

I have put out several job advertisements and I have received so many applicants. St George's Critical Care is on the map. Media coverage, CriticalNhs and the Duchess of Cambridge's *Hold Still* exhibition at the National Portrait Gallery have made us known. We have an excellent reputation, which, I think, is well deserved.

Nurses still want to be nurses – it's extraordinary, really.

We are still turning in circles, deciding if we are permanently increasing our Critical Care capacity. No decisions, and we joke about the new policy of the hour.

Everything in the NHS is connected to money and budgets. The unfathomable and blinkered logic of save money now, spend much more later. The false economy that has driven me crazy for years. The budgets that must be adhered to – never enough – and then the cutbacks.

We have strips running down the corridor floor to divide people traffic, and signs telling us to 'keep left' and remind us to social distance. Hand sanitiser dispensers have popped up everywhere and Pret have devised a one-way system, removing the tables and chairs where we would often meet and share a coffee with colleagues who became our friends.

I suspect we won't increase our bed capacity. We will surge, we will cope and we will do it all over again.

Resilience is in our DNA.

11 July

I was asked to say a few words at a local street event last Sunday, where there were celebrations and a clap to mark the seventy-second anniversary of the NHS. I didn't say much; what is there to say? Still words fail me, and I am someone who used to talk a lot.

I wasn't prepared for coronavirus and I hadn't prepared for this. 'If you know a nurse, particularly a Critical Care nurse, be kind to them, as we are all a little bit broken.'

The nation claps for the NHS, while others try to dismantle it. The NHS has been through the greatest test of its lifetime, and what now? Pubs are open yet it's impossible to book a non-urgent endoscopy, and my father, who is 88, cannot get an appointment to have his ears syringed.

We carry on regardless. The mix of different and often contradictory feelings continue for the staff. A close friend and senior colleague said, 'Life at the moment is like wearing wet socks. They are uncomfortable, you want to take them off. You get on with life, with work, chat with friends, do the regular stuff and appear normal, but are permanently distracted by wet socks. Talking, crying doesn't help – the socks are still wet.'

We remain, bruised, damaged, diminished.

I am lucky. I'm honoured and grateful to have an amazing family who support and love me unconditionally, no matter what or how wet my socks are. They wait for me as I untangle myself from the sticky Covid web.

On Wednesday I cared for a young patient following a massive stroke. Shocking for her family. A beautiful, vibrant woman, otherwise healthy, who had survived lockdown. Now all I can do is give her the best death I can. The rules have changed, and her family could see her and say goodbye. I felt a sadness for her, but also for all of our patients who died from coronavirus, whose family did not get to say goodbye. Sometimes an individual would be dropped off at A&E with a cough and a temperature, and never be seen again by the people who loved them. I hope you know that we always – as much as we possibly could – gave the very best care under extreme and hideous circumstances. No one died alone.

The hospital is beginning to resemble normal. The edges of the social-distancing stickers on the floor are beginning to lift. There is no red zone and, when I walked past our old Covid space, I could see regular staff and patients moving about just as they had before it all happened at the beginning of March.

Did it really happen? Did we live in a crazy, surreal bubble for just over three months, like being in the TV show *Stranger Things*, where monsters come out of the walls? I still see some memories played out in my dreams – when I am able to sleep.

Our nurses are bouncing back, laughing, chatting and planning holidays or a trip out. They post photos on social media of post-night-duty breakfast at a pub. The changing room is filled with shrieks of laughter, chat in different languages, in-jokes, playfulness, teasing. The strong camaraderie is born from what we shared together. Our powerful team. Bonded by an experience. How I missed this. These nurses, who not so long ago would change in this room in silence, with apprehension of their shift to come – or with exhaustion, when it came time to leave. Quiet and scared.

The days I went home with dried tears that had trickled into my ear, or make-up on my neck from those cuddles given to young nurses who would wrap themselves into me and sob. I would smell of different perfume as their scent attached itself to me. I am fond of these young women in a deep and lasting way. For many I was their backup mum, and I am proud of that role. Some of their real mums sent me messages or cards.

Surge or not? It doesn't seem to have happened yet. We have Covid fatigue and prefer to move forward. We are prepared for action but perhaps it won't happen. We will hit the ground running if it happens again. We have no extra staff, no extra beds. Talks of increasing our bed capacity have receded. Money – it's always about money.

Life goes on, as it should. But I, for one, will never quite be the same again. I will carry my Covid experience with me.

Not better, not worse. Just different.

20 July

My friend's mum said that waiting for my email is like looking forward to the next episode of *Killing Eve*.

I interviewed a Portuguese nurse who said, 'Covid shaped me, bent me, stretched me and scratched me.' That's a good way of putting it. Covid definitely scratched us all.

I am in charge today. Lots of trauma and lots of 'code red' – emergency jargon for massive haemorrhage. The Covid area was red. It's not like red for stop at the traffic lights: in our world red means go, go, go. It's definitely stepped up and is back to normal: the controlled and meticulous mayhem that is Critical Care. The more crazy it is, the more calm I feel. This is what I am trained to do.

The fog is lifting. This word-spew of observations and experience is not a cry for help. These are the rantings of a bruised Critical Care nurse who has used new-found skills of procuring food and excessive cuddling, and who has a propensity to show love and affection that is frequently rejected by my independent yet lovely 15-year-old son.

Hugs, biscuits and chocolate can't heal the world, but they really do make a difference. Social distancing is bad for the soul. People need to be with each other to thrive.

I have to delve into my bag to find yesterday's mask to walk through the door of the hospital or into an underground station. How is this good infection-control practice? The hospital observes and sets an example of current government guidelines, and I repeatedly see people don a filthy, well-used, flimsy mask, often used as a chin sling. So we adhere to the rules – but surely that cannot possibly help prevent the spread of Covid-19.

My emails continue to receive positive comment, though there are a few people – sometimes they have never met me – who remark critically on a specific example or story, with-out comment on the trauma we have experienced and are still unravelling from. I find this interesting and disturbing at the same time. Being kind must be how we are in order to move forward.

Please know that my patients always come first. They are the reason we do this. I do adjust situations, gender, the story – and I do this to ensure patient confidentiality. I create a generic persona. The staff are real and I always seek their permission, which they are willing to give. Our Trust is incredible, and light-hearted stories are only intended to paint a picture and a balance between real, reason and ridiculous.

It seems support and excellence come from the most unexpected places. I was fortunate enough to drink Prosecco in Tooting Market with a young but very wise Spanish nurse, and she helped nudge me back to reality. The younger nurses, of whom I have become so fond, constantly remind me that it's me who always supports them, so it is OK for it to be the other way round for a bit. I find this hard and uncomfortable as a team leader and senior sister, but in this crazy world things are still so back to front.

Claudia and I drove to see my parents. I had not seen them since early March and, as they are both in their eighties, I was worried about them. They are fine. On the three-hour drive back, we passed a recent nine-car pile-up on the motorway, with emergency vehicles in attendance. Some of the drivers and passengers might have ended up on Critical Care. I kept thinking about the incident. Since this viral menace invaded us, my empathy has increased a thousand-fold. I cannot bear to see anyone suffer. I have driven past many accidents before, stopping to help if needed. Now the rawness and knowledge of the profound impact this accident could have on an individual's life affects me with a new-found perspective. Before Covid, I took things for granted, but when it came it steered me to the darkest places and showed me my true self.

Covid patients are mostly home now. Families send us photos of them looking healthy. It's so rewarding to see. Some send cards or gifts and keep in touch. During the toughest times I would use my own phone to help patients communicate with their families; we all did. This is not permitted, advised or best practice, but extreme circumstances sometimes made it necessary. I noticed that not one family abused this or continued to call us. We just receive the odd message of thanks or a photo.

I have received many cards and messages from patients I've nursed. Some of them I don't remember, but mostly I can recall some part of their story. They wish us the best and say thank you.

I received an email from a young woman I nursed following a head-on car collision five years ago. She was not wearing a seatbelt, and her friend, who was driving the car, died. The young woman had a massive head injury and many broken bones. She just wanted to say hi by way of an email, and say thank you for what the staff are doing. She was fine, engaged to be married and, apart from being a bit stiff and forgetful, she had survived in every respect. Mostly, I remembered her mum, who sat by her daughter's bed, sobbing. She assumed her daughter would die, which was a very likely outcome at the time.

I love being a nurse; it is a part of who I am. Partner, mum, nurse, runner, friend and a 'fixer' in most situations. I know that, as the winter approaches, we will be busy again – always busy, frequently at capacity, but there are never enough staff or beds or equipment. Now the WHO reports the number of new daily infections worldwide has surpassed a quarter of a million. We just have to wait.

If you pass a hospital, drop off a box of biscuits – always appreciated and nurses can demolish a box of biscuits in seconds!

29 July

Swabs? It is so complicated for a fit and healthy, symptom-free nurse to get a Covid-19 swab. Government guidelines regarding travel have changed. Two negative swab results must be available, within five days prior to travel to some countries. But unless you have symptoms or have been in contact with a person with symptoms, it's not possible. Should we lie? We have been bathing in Covid. It should be celebrated that we survived this virus that killed so many. A simple swab is not asking much.

Team effort continues. Finally, the promotions have been approved. A few nurses are leaving but, interestingly, not because of the last few months. On my way to work I saw a slogan on the side of a red Routemaster bus: 'Great moments are the work of many.' The bus flew by, so I didn't catch what was being advertised or promoted, but we have made some great moments during the past crazy months. There was a great moment this week, when we were laughing at work so freely and easily; it was refreshing and a glimpse of the old normal.

Patients still stream in. Some as a result of having avoided a trip to hospital in fear of Covid during lockdown, while there are many more episodes of self-harm. Those who were struggling before lockdown were tipped over the edge with the isolation in our hug-free, mask-filled world. We had four motorbike accidents in one day; such a dangerous mode of transport, in my opinion.

London Scrubbers dropped off some fabric masks for me to distribute. All sizes and some for children. I took photos of the array of colourful choices and put them on our health-and-wellbeing WhatsApp group. I felt like an ice-cream lady, my phone pinging with requests for trains, dinosaurs, butterflies and green spots. Heads were popping around the office door, saying, 'I want the one with the rabbits, please.'

Many European nurses have returned from their trips home, tanned and rested, some with an added piercing or tattoo. I had been stalking them on Instagram, feeling so relieved to see them in the arms of family, where they had been desperate to be. Photos of beaches, mountains, pavement cafes, and Aperol spritz and mozzarella that have made my mouth water. I am very happy to now have Perugian salami in my fridge!

One Italian nurse confided in me that she felt displaced after a trip home. Covid had unnerved her. She was happy to be home at last in Italy, but also felt she needed to be in London. She was eager to be with her family where she belonged, yet where did she belong now?

We desperately need more Critical Care beds, despite Covid. We rarely have empty beds – patient flow is important. Once deemed fit for discharge from Critical Care and an appropriate bed is available, one patient is out, and shortly another patient is admitted – into a clean bed space, where the floor is mopped, the area cleaned and restocked and fresh linen put on the bed, ready for the next person who requires our care and perspective. However, there has not been one single Covid-related death at St George's for five weeks now. Perhaps the decision will be made the moment we surge and then we conjure it all up in a day – as before.

I cannot possibly comment on the fact that we are not one of the groups who will receive a pay rise. The nation clapped every Thursday for us but now we feel the clap has become a slap. Our hard work and resilience during the pandemic are now forgotten. We feel insulted and this demonstrates the total lack of understanding for what nurses have actually been through.

We worked so hard during the pandemic, and social distancing is impossible when you are caring for a ventilated patient or taking blood. You can't wash a dead body via Skype. You cannot empty a drainage bag over Zoom. CPR during a Microsoft Teams meeting is impossible. We put ourselves out there, on the line, over the line, and with no pay rise or bonus.

We are prepared to do it all again.

I ran 25 kilometres today. It was hot and hard work, but still nothing in comparison with a 12-hour shift in PPE at the height of the pandemic.

AUGUST 2020

4 August

We marinated in Covid for such a long time, and the debrief sessions we have each week are run by one of our fabulous team leaders. These gatherings are a chance for us to wallow in our memories of our trip to outer space. From cleaner to consultant, we all have a story to tell, each from a different perspective. A senior consultant said, 'I am old, fat and hypertensive, and I was really scared when I came to work.'

It's cathartic to know that we all feel the same. We can't sleep; Covid-lag, I call it. This week the most I slept in a night was five hours, and usually I sleep three to four hours a night. I don't feel tired, though: there is the adrenaline rush that I try to burn off when I run. Scratch the surface and we remain a bit emotional. It feels like a dream. The younger nurses are like a bouncy ball and are on the way up.

The future is complex and uncertain. We cannot predict what will be next. We are not on the front line anymore. The mask-wearing, hand-washing, social-distancing new population are on the front line; they control our future. We are on the back line, ready to catch you if you fall.

An Irish nurse said, 'It's OK to feel weird,' and perhaps it is. My axis has been tipped. My partner and I have just watched *Trigonometry*, an eight-part BBC series. It was brilliant, a welcome escape. My new perspective on life, my altered axis, enabled me to appreciate this superb British drama on another level. People are important, as is love and friendship.

A young man hanged himself. I spoke with the senior nurse for organ donation (SNOD) after his wife agreed for his organs to be donated. The senior nurse, who is also my friend, was finding it so hard. How do you support someone who has lost their husband, the father of their small children, in such a violent way? Nurses do so much more than anyone understands, and then even more on top of that. My friend had to tell the children, 'The doctors and nurses tried to make Daddy better, but they couldn't, so he died.'

There is no training for this. You learn it and find it from within yourself. We never get used to the heartache; we just find a place for it. This is someone else's story and grief, but if one day an individual looks back at the horrendous and traumatic experience of losing someone they love and a nurse made a difference, then that is enough. The messages I received during March, April and May showed me what a difference we make to our patients and their loved ones.

Many Spanish hearts are broken. These nurses worked through Covid and they now go home to see family, a new niece or nephew, attend their school friend's wedding, see an elderly relative. However, they must self-isolate for 14 days on their return, using their own annual leave or by taking unpaid leave. This makes me angry. I understand government Foreign Commonwealth Office (FCO) guidelines have changed, but can't we just support them? Why do we treat nurses so badly? They either cancel their trip or they leave. One of them said, 'I just want to hug my grandmother. That's what I want most.' No pay rise, no real gratitude, no bonus, no support. We go abroad to recruit nurses, yet this is how we repay them after what they have done. I feel ashamed.

A patient collapsed at the airport. The drugs he swallowed, wrapped in clingfilm to smuggle into the country, had burst inside him. A man jumped from a motorway bridge to end his life, and a woman chose to stop the treatment for her cancer. All patients on Critical Care; all desperate in their own way. Our medical team patch them up, relieve their pain and try to comfort their family. No salary can reward this brilliance.

The trajectory still heads towards normal, as normal as a day on Critical Care can ever be. We are actively recruiting new staff to train and mould into Critical Care nurses. Some of these nurses came to help during the pandemic and are now drawn to the madness and our supportive team. If there is a surge in coronavirus then at least we are already expanding our staff numbers.

The patients' bathroom has been fixed. Days of tolerating drilling and banging and sticky paper on the corridor floor and – *voilà!* A new bathroom that looks identical to the last one, with a minimal amount spent to refresh it and stop the leak. (I told a friend and colleague that the sticky paper on the floor was to catch rats. She believed me. 'Really?' she said. It goes to show that a Critical Care nurse is not fazed by anything.)

I keep writing. I continue to receive positive feedback and, in a weird way, I enjoy it now. It's cathartic to commit my brain fog to words. The crazy, funny, glorious madness that is Critical Care.

Please, please, tell your family what you want if you die. Would you donate your organs? Do you want to survive no matter what? Do you want to be ventilated to prolong your life if there is no chance of recovery? Would you want CPR?

Mostly we are fit and healthy, so this is not an issue, but then there is sudden illness or traumatic injury or, as we get older ...

Our family need to know our wishes but rarely do. If they do, it makes it just a little bit easier.

9 August

The R factor is steady. It's the reproductive number that suggests the ability of the disease to spread. We remain surge-free in London at least, with the R factor currently at 0.8. It's taken a monumental effort to reduce this number through lockdown and social distancing.

The world has changed. We used to shake hands. Traditionally, we used to offer our empty right hand to show we meant no harm, a way of showing a stranger that we were not holding a weapon. Now we don't shake another person's hand for fear of causing them harm. This damages morale, and a stranger recoiling from me in the bread aisle in Sainsbury's makes me feel sad. How will our future be?

I am bouncing back, slowly, floating to the surface. The junior nurses who were instrumental in fixing me introduced me to the pleasure of Aperol spritz and I will never look back. A drink the colour of sunshine that will always remind me of Italian and Spanish awesomeness, eyeliner and lipstick.

I received a message from a nurse who left. She should have departed for her new job in April but stayed on for the storm. 'Thank you for all those moments of kindness and nonsense.'

Critical Care is like no other place, impossible to describe to those who do not work there. What happens behind those walls is bizarre and incredible. Often sad, often phenomenal and often hilarious. When I leave work after a clinical shift and walk up Tooting High Street to go home, I often think, *If you had any idea what I did today ...*

Trust plays a huge part in our care. Anxiety is amplified during an illness or accident. Patients are exposed. Always wearing their worst pants and, if they are lucky, they are aware enough to realise. Sometimes we get to know the intimate details of a person's life in minutes, leaving them exposed and vulnerable, but we respect this, and anything shared remains with us. We can keep secrets. Once I steered out a wife after visiting so that the long-term girlfriend could visit. One not knowing about the other.

I remember a young girl, just home from travelling in Kenya. She had a fabulous tan, with white marks that outlined her bikini. She became acutely unstable very fast – whatever African infection had overwhelmed her young, healthy body was rapidly beating her. Her mum witnessed us performing CPR on her daughter. No parent should have to experience this. She developed multiple pneumothoraces (life critical damage to the lungs, causing gas to accumulate in the pleural spaces, blowing up like a balloon with every breath, progressively squashing vital organs including the lungs and heart). The treatment? A chest tube, the diameter of a Malteser, is inserted between the ribs. She required seven chest tubes, and two Critical Care doctors inserted these simultaneously, efficiently and quickly to support her breathing, but they kept to the white areas of her otherwise tanned chest. The irony, as this 21-year-old girl was probably going to die.

She didn't die. Weeks later, when she was awake and had a tracheostomy to support her breathing, I helped her to have a wash. She wrote on a piece of paper, 'Did my mum pack my make-up?!'

She sent a postcard the following year from Australia. She had just won a tennis match and was off for a run on the beach.

These patients stay with me. Their survival makes us continue, no matter what. When she wears her bikini no one can see her scars. Some patients wear their scars with pride. A man who lost his wife and both legs in a motorbike accident came back to visit with his prosthetic legs. One had flashing lights, flock wallpaper and a Nike trainer. The other leg sported a brown leather brogue with a 'hairy' leg and purple and green stripes.

'I thought I might as well go for it,' he said.

A young girl fell under a Tube train. She was with a friend, messing about on the platform. She had horrendous and life-changing injuries, yet she survived. One day, years later, I bumped into her and asked, 'How did you deal with it?'

'I have two choices,' she told me. 'I either get over it or I don't.'

The patients are often our inspiration. There are those who rise up despite everything. And some simply give up, having acquired various health problems in life. There are those who embrace being unwell or being elderly, and seem to relish being dependent.

I will never part from independence and the desire to be a free spirit, particularly since my axis on life has tipped. People are incredible and loving makes everything possible – so it should. We keep on going.

I continue to forget my mask. I am pretty sure they don't make any difference, but mask-wearing is a mark of respect for others. So I must and will comply. I just have to remember!

*   *   *

Throughout the hottest and most humid August in the late nineties, when I was doing my Critical Care course, which was then called the ENB 100 (English National Board), I worked on the cardiac ICU. When you look out of the window just outside the current Cardiothoracic Critical Care, you can see the remains of Wright Ward. Back then it was where cardiac surgery and heart and lung transplants were performed, and it was home to the dialysis unit.

Now the diggers consume the earth where the building once stood. A vast abandoned space that once saw so much. The London stock bricks are cleaned to be sold and only a solitary cherry tree remains. Staff would often congregate on their break and have a smoke and chat and laugh under that tree.

On the first day my mentor asked me to outline my objectives. I remembered a night shift in A&E in my final year as a student, when a young man was admitted with multiple stab wounds. A cardiothoracic surgeon was called, as this man was bleeding profusely. I watched in amazement as he performed an emergency thoracotomy (making an incision in the chest wall between the ribs). The surgeon inserted his hand into the open chest and performed internal cardiac massage as we tried to replace the lost blood.

It was Christmas, and there was blood all over the floor. The sparkle of silver tinsel and the ribbons of coloured paper sprinkled into the blood, festive decorations that had fallen from staff who had adorned their stethoscopes or hair to mark the season; this is an image that has remained with me.

Another surgeon tried to stem the blood flow and patch up the damage so that the patient could be taken to theatre for a definitive repair. This was exciting and I was drinking in the information and experience, noting such calm in this vivid emergency. I was learning so much. When I started working on the cardiac unit, I wanted to see a procedure where the chest was opened. To see the heart and lungs exposed is a true anatomy lesson.

My objectives outlined, my mentor assured me that I would definitely see them 'crack a chest'. If a post-operative patient on the cardiac unit had a cardiac arrest, their chest would be re-opened, the wires holding the sternum together cut and internal cardiac massage and defibrillation performed, far superior than standard CPR. Wright Ward had a great reputation for cardiac surgery, and I knew that it was a truly remarkable place to work. The nurses were fabulous, and I still work with one of them today.

I learned so much over the next few weeks. I wrote my essays and learning plan. I completed my pre-set competencies. And I loved it, caring for people after major heart surgery performed by world-renowned cardiac surgeons. I learned how to care for patients following their elective cardiac surgery, and how to progress their recovery so that they were fit enough to be discharged to the ward. I nursed people who had an OOHCA (out of hospital cardiac arrest). Some would make a full recovery after a procedure to fix the problem. On my final day, I took in a large tin of homemade biscuits to say thank you for all the support and teaching (nurses always default to cake and biscuits).

I had a fascinating few weeks, but I had not seen an open chest on my shift. It would always happen on the shift before or the next shift. 'It was amazing,' my colleagues would say. 'Incredible.' But I kept missing it. And then ...

My final shift was on a Friday. At the end of the day I changed into my clothes and walked off the ICU saying, 'No open chest.' The nurses laughed and waved me off.

'Anthea!' My mentor screamed my name. I turned back and walked down the corridor as fast as I could – was this an open chest? 'No,' my mentor said. 'Put scrubs on, eat something, have a drink and do a wee – quickly.'

I had no idea what was happening. I put my bag in the locker, did what I was told and phoned home to say I might be late.

My mentor handed me a large blue cool box and said, 'Go down the ramp and get into the car.' I had absolutely no idea what we were doing, but I was pretty sure we weren't going on a picnic. Down the ramp and through the heavy door … and there was a white emergency-response vehicle with an orange and blue stripe and flashing lights. The doors and boot were wide open.

My cool box was taken from me and put into the boot. Three more people appeared in scrubs. We all got into the car and were told to fasten our seat belts.

This was exciting. I asked what was happening as the car pulled out of the hospital, lights and sirens on, and we took off at rollercoaster speed, zooming down Blackshaw Road, through Wimbledon and weaving through the streets of south-west London, as traffic moved aside to let us pass. We flew through red lights – I still had no idea what was happening – and in no time at all we were on the M4.

Once we were doing 100 mph on the motorway – I was straining my eyes to see the speedometer – I was told that we were going to France to collect some lungs. I was in the car with the organ transport retrieval team, who were going to remove the lungs from a French teenager who was now brain dead following a traffic accident. The lungs were for a young woman at St George's. This was surreal. This was my open-chest moment.

We drove directly onto the runway at Heathrow and hurriedly boarded an RAF Learjet, and took off for Montpellier, in the south of France. As soon as the jet was in the sky the team put their seats back and went to sleep. I was buzzing. They were not very chatty and were super chilled, as they were regulars at this.

'Your first time?' said the pilot.

We landed in France and a dilapidated ambulance tore through the streets of Montpellier at midnight, over cobbled streets, twisting and turning while I clutched my cool box. We arrived at a hospital where the doors were held open by staff awaiting our arrival. We were directed to the operating theatre, where there were other teams already present to retrieve this young man's heart or liver or kidneys. The young donor was on the operating table, his internal organs exposed. The removal of various organs by experts was controlled, remarkable and respectful. There is a process and an order in which organs are removed.

Once the lungs were ready for removal, the ventilator that had been providing oxygen was turned off. The young man lay open. He was giving the gift of life to five other people. Organ donation is an incredible thing and the only positive to come from a person's death.

The lungs were removed from the donor, inflated with oxygen, packed on ice and placed inside my cool box. We returned to the airport and in no time at all we were in the air, heading back to London to transplant the lungs into the recipient, who I later learned had been on the waiting list for three months.

The team went to sleep again, and now I realised why. They were required to perform two operations, in two different countries, within hours of each other. This required skill, knowledge, experience and the ability to stay alert and focused for the double lung transplant.

I had never felt more awake. I was invited into the cockpit and that is where I stayed until we landed at 5 a.m. We flew above the Thames, over London, towards Heathrow. I looked down on Big Ben and the Houses of Parliament as the sun was rising on yet another hot and glorious day. It was truly magnificent.

We arrived at St George's in record time. The recipient was ready, her fibrosed lungs visible in her open chest. She was on cardiopulmonary bypass (a technique in which a machine temporarily takes over the function of the heart and lungs during surgery).

The team scrubbed up again and her lungs were replaced with the young healthy ones. I watched as they were placed in her chest, connected to her blood vessels and arteries, and the ventilator breathed in and out. Pressure settings on the ventilator immediately reduced, as these healthy lungs were functioning well. Her discarded, unhealthy, exhausted lungs were placed on a metal tray, now redundant.

I visited the patient a few days later on a cardiac ward. She was young and chatty, and said that she felt fantastic despite recovering from major surgery. She told me that she hadn't been able to walk more than ten metres, climb stairs or complete a sentence as she was so breathless, and she was dependent on being given oxygen. Now she was laughing and chatting and so happy, without the oxygen.

'The surgeon told me I have French lungs,' she said, and laughed.

I got my open chest. I learned so much that night, and to this day it remains one of the most memorable experiences of my life. Slick and superb, all of this was for one person. Someone died and someone could go on to live a full life again.

In these situations, despite the excitement and awesomeness, I knew there was a family in France who had been devastated, as someone they loved had died. However, they had also made a decision that would offer other people a chance to live.

16 August

The weather is glorious. The sun lifts our spirits. It's tricky for the nurses working night shifts to sleep during the day while it is so hot and humid. Night shifts leave you feeling jet-lagged, disorientated and a bit sick. I haven't worked a night shift for years. I was supposed to work a few when Covid exploded, but a wonderful Filipino nurse worked them for me and I worked her day shifts (many lovely nurses offered to work the night shifts for me, as they know I don't deal well with them at all).

Portuguese nurses are going home now. I love Portugal and we often go to Tavira, in the Algarve. I found it hilarious when a nurse asked me about places to visit and said that the Portuguese nurses had suggested she ask my advice, as I know the Algarve better than them. We often act as one another's travel advisory service. I want to be on the beach in Portugal and eat a warm doughnut filled with the yellow, creamy custard bought from one of the tanned Portuguese sellers who walk back and forth along the seafront with a basket of these delicious delights, calling out, 'Bolinha!'

Bravery, grit and love is how a friend described my musings about Critical Care nursing. From her perspective, it was good to learn about the reality of what happens behind the doors – the doors that don't work properly, with the sensor that sometimes responds and often not, meaning that one door has to be wedged open sometimes, and the other door randomly closes at the worst moment, all while a bed and all the kit need to be moved swiftly down the corridor. The doors in Sainsbury's, Waitrose and Lidl never have this issue. I am sure their doors also deal with the odd customer who is sometimes a bit too rough.

We were hit by a tsunami and now the wave is in the distance, but some of the floating rubble remains. It's hard to reflect. We have no memory of those times really, except of being there and going through the process. My father said, 'It must be like riding a bicycle that wobbles, trying to keep going and not fall off.' It is a bit, but we did fall off and we mostly got straight back on.

Now it is different things that are stressful. A nurse opened her fridge and realised she had run out of yoghurt, which caused her to cry for hours.

We continue to bond. If we see someone we recognise in the corridor, someone who helped during the rage, we are able to identify them from their eyes because that's how we saw each other during that time because of the PPE. Our eyes connect us. We know, and we did it together.

We refer to our journey to outer space, or somewhere else that has no meaning or reality, which we still can't grasp or understand. It's changed many of us. It's definitely changed me.

The alchemy of Critical Care staff is always superb. I worked with my team the other day and a patient suddenly deteriorated; she stopped breathing. Another ICU nurse, a physiotherapist and I did what we do best – used our knowledge, skills, experience and training to reverse the issue, addressing the problem in a calm and competent manner, and with a huge group of new junior doctors looking on in amazement. 'Feel free to help,' I said. They snapped into action, awoken from their side-line view, and offered their help, but by then the issue was resolved and a new junior doctor began issuing instructions that we had already fulfilled. Even after Covid some staff forget that the Critical Care nurses are geniuses.

I received a WhatsApp message today. It read simply: 'Madrid'. Meaning that one of my Spanish nurses had put her Spanish feet on Spanish soil to breathe Spanish air. This same nurse described Covid like this: 'I don't have many memories from that period. I was just going to work. I was trying to keep the patients alive until the next shift. That was it. Just keep them alive.'

Usually, she returns home every two to three months, but due to Covid this is her first trip home in eight months. I love how they let me know when they arrive home – it's a 'Mummy' thing.

We need more Critical Care beds; we need more nurses. We needed this before the pandemic and we will need extra capacity after the pandemic in order to catch up with abandoned elective surgery and the casualties of Covid, as well as the regular stream of sick and injured patients. Never enough money or resources or beds – not actually the bed but the space for the bed. I frequently joke that we should order bunk beds from IKEA – anyone with diarrhoea should be on the bottom bunk!

A new Critical Care unit will cost millions of pounds, and where would this be built in a huge hospital that has so little space to spare?

A sneaky night out with friends ended in disaster for a young man who thought some experimental drug-taking would be fun. His life will never be the same again, as he had a reaction resulting in him requiring major surgery. It reminded me why I am so antirecreational drug use. Most people get away with it, have fun and are oblivious as to how it affects them long-term. Some don't get away with it at all and it destroys their lives.

Next week I am interviewing junior staff – some of the applications are from support nurses who helped us during the pandemic's surge. There have been more applicants than ever, which surprised me – I really thought there would be fewer. But no, more incredible people want to board the crazy train. It's exciting, as I know that we will recruit some amazing people to add to our eclectic mix of fabulousness.

I had coffee in Pret with two young ICU nurses, one of them Italian, the other Spanish. We shared recollections. The Spanish nurse is 'a little bit scared' that it will happen again, that there'll be another wave and more hospitalisations. But she is proud of the role she has played, and rightly so. 'I have been part of something really big and important. I did my bit. And we did our best. Sometimes I think about the ones who died. Then you see all the patients we saved and people clapping, and I feel proud. And now when I go round the hospital, even though we are all wearing these masks, I can recognise these people from other wards in the hospital just from their eyes. And I'm like, "Hey, how are you?" I feel comfortable with those people.'

She is coping well. 'I can compartmentalise,' she says. 'I never bring anything home. What happens in the hospital, happens in the hospital.'

'I am like a yo-yo,' I said to them. 'I seem all right, and then one tiny thing and whoosh – I'm in tears and I don't know why.'

Unless the FCO government travel advice changes, my next epistle will be penned from the beach in Italy.

I salute our nurses. They are incredible, brave and resilient, and so much fun.

24 August

It's Claudia's last week at St George's. Who could have imagined that we would work together in such a way? What a phenomenal and life-changing experience for her, one that has united us on yet another level. After almost six months of Covid-19 pandemic support, she has left, and her departure is accompanied by many jokes from my cheeky colleagues: 'Can't she stay and you go?' She got a great send-off, with cards, gifts, pizza and a trip to the pub.

There was a young patient who tried to kill herself, jumping off a building. But instead of ending her life, she caused herself life-long injuries. She has been in hospital so long and undergone so many different surgeries that I think she has forgotten why she was admitted in the first place. Long-term hospital-ised patients become institutionalised to the point that it is scary for them to leave. They become unwittingly dependent on the routine and endless stream of people involved in their care. This is now their life. The rehabilitation journey is long, arduous and challenging.

Thank you can never be enough. No pay rise, no bonus, nothing to recognise what we did and what we may need to do again.

The Saffir-Simpson Hurricane Wind Scale is used to rank hurricanes on a scale of one to five, depending on the wind speed. The wind speed of Covid-19 hit a scale that does not exist. We need some form of remuneration to acknowledge the wind speed we experienced.

Nurses take their holiday time to quarantine when return-ing from Europe. All 'non-essential travel' is not encouraged. I think that being with your family after the last few months is essential travel, on every level. Nurses are, as usual, on the back foot.

Winter is always busy in Critical Care, so some nurses have been refused time off at Christmas. If we have a surge on top of the usual winter pressures it will be hard to manage, but we will be expected to do it, without fuss, without reward, regard-less of our own personal circumstances.

Social distancing means keeping apart from people to restrict the spread of coronavirus. Keeping apart from people is also bad for our mental health. We have been advised to minimise contact and mixing: something so important that quenches the soul. Some people enjoy the space, the excuse not to embrace or have to meet up with someone. For me, social and tactile, I find it abhorrent, sad and wrong on many levels.

I have received gifts from my nurses' mums this week. They say thank you for supporting their daughters. I love being the back-up surrogate mum for these lovely young nurses. I love their messages filled with affection, and the hugs that I receive, the requests for advice or support. I cherish the pastoral aspect of my work that has always been there, and it brings out the best in me. This role, and the need for this role, has increased exponentially over the last few months and hasn't changed, even though things are more settled now.

St George's admitted a few Covid-positive patients this week. We are alert. Is this it? Do we board the Covid Express once more?

Our unit remains quiet. Patients, following emergency or elective surgery, used to trickle in daily. There are new rules in theatres to prevent virus transmission and maintain patient safety, and therefore surgery is limited. There must be a backlog of those having to wait longer. And as Critical Care admits patients following major surgery, I am concerned that their wait time will contribute to their health deterioration.

Staff have spent time cleaning and organising equipment. The store room, empty a few months ago, now looks organised, polished and efficient. Machinery is now plentiful – waiting for the next victim.

Italy is everything it promised. It is so good to lie on the beach in the sun, the mozzarella is out of this world and the Aperol spritz refreshing and relaxing. A beautiful country in which to recharge and regroup, and I have the added bonus of Italian translation, advice and suggestions just a WhatsApp click away. All my Italian nurses and friends are keen to support and advise me.

An elderly man misses his wife; there are still restrictions for visitors. 'She's as annoying as hell. But I would rather be annoyed by her than not see her at all.' FaceTime communication via iPad has been an amazing communication method for patients and their families over the past months. It's not the same as face-to-face, of course, but it's OK until we can allow family and friends to visit once more.

This pandemic has taught us that the people we love are important. This matters above everything and we need to find our purpose and pursue it relentlessly.

The helicopter still lands, the ambulances still arrive. There is a socially distanced queue outside our emergency department (formally A&E, now ED – who knows why this was changed). Patients arrive to be fixed, reassured, treated. The NHS is amazing and should be preserved at all costs.

My lilo beckons. I have spent hours floating on the water, dozing, relaxing, tanning. I ran 20 kilometres yesterday morning along the beach and coastal path. The sun and running – my two favourite happy places.

30 August

A few weeks ago I recruited 18 new junior nurses. One nurse said at her interview that helping on Critical Care during the pandemic was like being in a rain shower without an umbrella. For my team, it felt like we were pelted with rocks by Dementors: no shelter, no defence and certainly no rain!

A 58-year-old woman was admitted with high blood pressure. So high and uncontrolled that she had headaches, saw flashing lights and had collapsed at Gatwick Airport after returning from a three-month stay with her sister in St Lucia. She had recently been put on medication for her newly elevated blood pressure, but the pills gave her nausea and indigestion. She was exhausted, so she had taken a break from her stressful, high-powered job to relax and spend time with family, gaining weight due to rest and the abundance of delicious West Indian food. I looked after her the morning she was admitted to Critical Care.

It was a student nurse who saw it first. There it was – the undeniable visual movement, just as I had experienced myself during pregnancy. Little prods from feet and elbows against the abdominal wall, the fidgeting foetus awake and wriggling around in the uterus. An ultrasound revealed a full-term baby, who was promptly removed by emergency caesarean. The baby was causing an acute deterioration in the mother's health and roared into the world having caused pre-eclampsia disguised as high blood pressure. A woman in her fifties, the patient had presumed menopause, weight gain and wind, not pregnancy, despite all her pregnancy-related symptoms. Her husband and adult children were so shocked. I think her son was more disturbed that his mother was sexually active than he was at learning that he had a new sibling.

Once my patient was awake but still intubated (a breathing tube in place), we explained what had happened. She looked horrified. Then she smiled, shrugged her shoulders and pointed at her breasts.

I explained, 'Yes, you can breast feed. Once you are more awake and the sedation has worn off, I'll remove the breathing tube so that you can talk.' The baby was fine, being examined by the midwives on the maternity unit. The baby weighed 3 kilograms and was healthy. The mother, meanwhile, kept pointing at her abdomen and trying to mouth words that I couldn't understand. I did all I could to reassure her.

I asked if she wanted to write down the question that was bothering her. She nodded and then wrote the best thing: 'Boy or girl?' In all the madness and trying to explain the situation and reassure her, not one of us had told her that she had a new son. It was wonderful to see the connection between mother and baby. She kissed him all over his little face and then connected him to her breast like a pro. Not a usual sight on Critical Care, but perfect in that moment.

The tinnitus of busy goes on. The agony of illness for some, who are with us until we aid their recovery or ensure they have a good death – dignified and in comfort. The patients are admitted from ED (the name change discussed in my last email), the wards or theatres, or as an emergency. Our outreach team scoop up and rescue a deteriorating adult and bring them to us, efficiently and in a timely manner. Hopefully we have a spare empty bed and a nurse available. Many patients are admitted, fixed and discharged home to continue with their life.

Weeks ago I mentioned a patient who had suffered badly from the metabolic and psychotic effects of recreational drug use. Now that patient has recovered, and he came back to say hello. It's extraordinary and I have sometimes shed a tear when a patient returns to say hello or thank you. They often have no memory of their stay on Critical Care, or they just remember something random or the voice of a particular member of staff.

Covid crazy continues. Meticulous but daft rules. In Italy our temperatures were taken before going onto the beach, and on a boat by a man wearing a mask under his nose. I saw a woman wearing a mask in the sea and a young man who pushed his mask down when he sneezed. I saw an elderly lady in Balham use a disinfectant spray cleaner and J Cloth to clean the ATM machine, and then she adjusted her mask with her gloved hands.

Wash your hands, don't touch your face or mask, and change your towels daily.

I return to work this week after a wonderful holiday, where the water was turquoise and the food was amazing. Happy to return and mostly recovered now from whatever it was that happened to me and to my colleagues

There are still no words.

SEPTEMBER 2020

6 September

Back to work after a superb holiday with my fantastic family. Lunch with one of my favourite people on the South Bank; running miles and miles, and suddenly the weird place is fading. I am more me and back to happy. As I have said before, my axis has altered. The rage train has, in the end, given me strength, courage and hope. It's OK to cry, to be sad and to feel overwhelmed. It's also OK to accept support from wherever feels best.

Despite our age, we do change and grow, and this is a good thing. I have learned some tough, incredible and marvellous lessons over the last six months; lessons about love, friendship and camaraderie, and how extraordinary it is. Luckily, despite everything, I have retained my sense of humour throughout this strange time.

I love the work I do, and no matter what implodes I will be there. Many of my wonderful work colleagues feel the same. I am a nurse through to my bones. We embrace the chaos, the busy, the madness – the everyday that is Critical Care. And when I arrive at work, I have no idea what the day will bring. We are precise, there is attention to detail, yet we face constant unpredictability. I embrace that balance. We can be immersed in suffering and celebration all at the same time.

A man had a tumour in his mouth, a lump on his jaw discovered just before lockdown and ignored. It is now resected, and his jaw reconstructed by a brilliant maxillofacial surgeon who took six hours to take bone, tissue and muscle from the man's thigh and hip to rebuild his jaw. Once he was awake, I asked, 'Are you in pain?'

'No, not really. Did it rain today?'

Magnificent happens at St George's in many ways but there is a great deal of ridiculous. Claudia has been asked to attend an induction day, having already finished her six months' work on Critical Care. She will be paid to do this induction course. She relayed a bizarre conversation to me that she had with the person who made the booking – a waste of time and money from the NHS's already near-empty purse. But ... 'It's policy.'

Discussions about expansion continue. The details change daily as different healthcare professionals update the team on the current plan from their perspective. I recently walked along the corridor and was given the same information three times but with three different final outcomes. Needless to say, we have no idea what the plan is. But once a final – final – decision is made, we will jump to attention and do what we need to do, always delivering the best care possible. You can be sure that whatever plan is made there will be the same old caveat and there will be a lot of furniture, beds and equipment moving around.

Currently we have three patients at the end of their lives, from illness and accident. Their families may now visit for short, pre-arranged periods. Visitors can be tricky: emotionally overwrought, shocked, upset, frustrated, guilty. Sometimes these emotions are expressed angrily, and are frequently directed at the nurses, who calmly and kindly try to explain and reassure honestly and openly. A few people do not have the vocabulary to express their true feelings, and this is when they can become rude, aggressive and, on occasion, violent.

Our pregnant consultant was punched in the stomach; another doctor was punched in the face. And a man held his face so close to mine while he demanded information I was not at liberty to share that I could feel his spit on my face as he growled at me. This was pre-Covid, luckily.

A few families think it's OK to be abrupt or rude to staff. They think their grief and shock justifies their behaviour. I have been told to 'fuck off' or 'shut up'. I understand that it rips your heart out to lose someone you love. We see the pain in loss. The guilt in some, as their last interaction with the patient might not have been ideal or they might not have seen them for a long time; the dismay, disbelief and all-consuming sadness.

But it hurts, it's humiliating and we never receive an apology. We never retaliate; we take the verbal punches and tolerate the abuse. I remember a father calling me a 'stupid bitch' and dragging his seven-year-old son kicking and screaming through ICU, insisting he kiss his dying mother goodbye. The boy did not recognise the septic patient connected to tubes and machines as his mother. He was terrified. He did not want to kiss the mound in the bed. I wondered if this small boy would suffer for life from this experience. I gently suggested to the father that if his son said he didn't want to see his mummy, perhaps he shouldn't be made to. He could draw a picture to give her instead.

Recently a family did not agree with visiting restrictions during Covid. To them, their family member transcended government guidelines and hospital policy. Their family member was more important than our other patients who had been denied visitors during the pandemic. Currently the hospital policy is this: long-term patients may have two visitors, twice a week; those who are dying may have two visitors; those who are initially admitted to our unit may have two visitors. This family had one member who was not open to reason and thought being rude and aggressive and insulting to me would achieve their desired outcome.

Some individuals can be intimidating but staff unite as a team to support each other. We recognise that their internal pain is overwhelming. Some people shout and scream admonishing expletives. Punching the wall, kicking the chair or being rude to the staff is how they release their hurt and frustration.

Sometimes we develop a deep bond with a family that lasts while the patient is in our care. We connect and communicate with family, and it's always a shock and uncomfortable for staff to deal with those who are not open to this temporary but very special relationship, particularly with the Critical Care nurses, who spend the entire day and night with the families' loved ones.

Some families cannot decide who is the next of kin, or the next of kin is estranged. Families may feel they get to approve or agree the care for an unconscious patient. Treatment or not, any decision is always made by the medical team in the individual patient's best interests.

Recently there was an issue when a severely injured motor-bike-accident victim required surgery. The family were informed the day before and then surgery was cancelled because he was too unstable. This did not make sense to them. They understood that the surgery was vital. The minute-by-minute decisions made in this environment are unsettling for loved ones, especially when the plan changes. They felt that the information was conflicting.

We always do our best to communicate as openly as we can. Most families are, of course, incredible and lovely, and we develop a close link in a matter of moments: the barriers are broken and we see their true selves. They express their grief in a tangible way. They cry, they accept comfort and kindness. We are used to supporting devastated and shocked families.

Many families we knew from years ago sent messages of gratitude and support during Covid. It takes a special person to empathise, support and connect, developing an instant rapport with a family. We want to ensure that, when they look back, they remember that the nurses were kind. The best comment is: 'You made such a difference.' And we do.

The office was a tip. After a tidy up we found all the missing pieces of paper, the Sellotape, my headphones and a box of Walkers salt and vinegar crisps stashed under a desk. Thirty bags of crisps. They were gone in moments. Who knew nurses could eat crisps so fast?

I'm not a technophobe but, unlike anyone under the age of 30, I can't text using both thumbs simultaneously – I watch in awe and astonishment. These young IT-savvy whizz-kids save me, solving my technical issues at work in moments. I love working with a younger generation who are fun and brilliant, and the IT Covid support team (uni students drafted in to help) were a breath of fresh air. It was a total honour to be included in their evenings out and shenanigans. I have learned about Instagram at last, Outlook and iPhone shortcuts. Already I miss them now that they have finished with us, though I am embarrassed to say that I still message or call them when I get stuck.

I'd better get this email sent. I now receive messages asking where my weekend email is. A cup of tea and my email – who ever would have thought it? I always like to chat and tell a story, and now I write them down.

15 September

Another trip out with my junior team to a bar in Tooting Market. I had said I wouldn't go but was persuaded by Italian pleading. Over Prosecco, some of the nurses reminded me of a day in April, when we were shattered after a particularly stressful and challenging shift. We had doffed our PPE and said goodbye. I needed to share a few details with the nurse in charge of the night shift, so it was 20 minutes later when I went into the coffee room to retrieve my bag. Nine nurses were sitting in the room: too tired to go home, too stressed to leave, needing to be with those who understood. We were in a weird place and it didn't feel right to go home. We needed a bonding trip to the pub but that was impossible, as it was at the height of lockdown.

I found a bottle of Pinot Grigio, given to me the week before. It was lukewarm from being in a bag under a chair. I opened it and each of us drank an inch of the pale-yellow liquid from cheap plastic cups. Some togetherness after the death and trauma of such a shift. A sip of warm wine tasted good, shared together in a scruffy, cramped coffee room, while sitting on uncomfortable sofas or rickety chairs under a flickering strip light. Those memories tap into our vulnerabilities and send a shiver down my spine, but also remind me why I was sitting in Tooting Market with an eclectic mix of awesome nurses.

Each electric wheelchair has its own system of working. Knobs, levers, a start and stop button. This chair was different.

It took four able-bodied, intelligent nurses to work out how to manoeuvre the chair, which seemed to be either stationary or fly off at 30 mph. There was much hilarity, but finally – after testing it out with each other whizzing around a Critical Care unit – it was parked by its owner's bed. A patient with a neuro-logical deficit who communicates only by using his eyes and a computer typed, 'They are all mad here!' His sense of fun shone through despite his limited communication abilities. A moment of humour shared – patient and nurses.

Tragedy happens in a diabolic way. To lose your unborn baby, your best friend, your partner, your mum and your dog – and you were the one driving – is more than any human should have to bear. There are no words to console or reassure. Often our patients are an inspiration and a reminder that our life is OK. If you end your day and everyone you hold close is alive and well, then it is enough. Since Covid, I find any suffering impossible to process. Even when watching some scenes on television I am covering my eyes. The contradiction of strength and fragility in a human being is phenomenal.

A recovered Covid patient came to visit, bringing cake and a massive bunch of sunflowers. Walking independently, his frail body had gained weight, and he looked brilliant considering that he'd almost died. So good to see him. He said that through his coma he felt as if he were on a space-ship or submarine – he absorbed the vibe well. So good to see our hard work pay off and that he remembered so many of us.

Covid patients are apparently increasing. The R factor is up. Critical Care have zero Covid patients. It seems those affected are not as sick as before. There are patients in Critical Care in smaller hospitals, and there has been talk about transferring them to us. So far, however, they remain where they are. The surge is seemingly less brutal, but we are ready. We can and will do it again and this time we are prepared. While the scientists aim to break the enigma code of Covid, so we wait to see if we are needed – ventilators calibrated, monitors charged and PPE on standby.

My recruitment role doubles up as a friendship agency. Nurses who do not know each other before coming to our Critical Care team then make some life-long bonds and close friendships. One of the hardest things during Covid was watching my colleagues struggle emotionally but just keep going. When I try to reflect on that time now it's so hard to recall, as it seems impossible. We were at war.

Four nurses and I helped move a patient to a different position. She weighed 210 kilograms (33 stone) and had poorly managed diabetes. She was unable to move independently due to her massive bulk. It was important to protect her skin and prevent pressure sores developing, so we adjusted her position every few hours. We needed a team to do this. During these Covid times there are not enough staff; it was difficult and any clinical staff available were summoned to help.

The patient was chatty and friendly, and before we repositioned her she asked me to pass her bottle of Coke so she could take a few sips. The Coke was on the overbed table, which was piled high with forbidden fruits – toffee, chocolate-covered raisins and a sherbet Dip Dab.

She offered us all a toffee and we then repositioned her comfortably on her side, wedging her in position with pillows and then elevating the head of her bed, as her weight compromised her breathing. I discussed the disadvantage of eating high-sugar snacks while trying to manage her blood-sugar levels. Lovely lady, but completely disengaged from her diabetes.

Turning any patients can create difficulties. There are drips and tubes and lines to mind and hold in place. Obese, cachectic, unstable patients or those in severe pain create another challenge. Those who have external metal work fixed in place to realign their bones, or some who have major wounds or unstable fractures. Any adjustment can cause something to dislodge or become disconnected. We turn people with an undiscussed precision, ensuring a patient is comfortable, protected and safe. Some patients may require a bolus of analgesia or sedation, and those who are awake often groan as they prefer not to be manhandled and we gently explain our rationale. If a person with capacity refuses to be turned, we respect their decision and try again later.

20 September

It's challenging when a patient is confused, often trying to climb out of bed or pulling at various tubes and monitoring leads. ICU delirium is a frequent issue, a fluctuating disturbance of consciousness and cognition. An acute brain dysfunction in critically ill patients.

Sometimes, when they finally succumb to sleep, lying sideways, hanging off the bed, tangled in sheets and wires, we leave them while they are calm. Anyone passing might frown, wondering why a patient is in such a state. A patient's agitation can be controlled with drugs, but these can often exacerbate the situation or cause other issues.

Some patients feel there is a conspiracy or that the government is controlling them. One patient didn't want to sleep in a car park, while another spent the day anxious about whether he had locked up the house properly. A few ask us to call the police. We do what we can to reassure them and keep them safe.

I had to see someone on the ward today – the ward that had been our temporary ICU at the peak of the pandemic. It's now a regular ward, and it was so odd and I felt tearful and emotional as I walked into that space. The space that had overwhelmed us when we were taken to another dimension. I felt heavy hearted for the rest of the day, memories of that time ignited. We are still healing, it seems.

*　　*　　*

Precise communication with patients is important and can make a huge difference. Nurses always pay attention to detail. It's the detail that can make the difference.

A few years ago I had a patient who had hit his head while cycling. He had glanced at his phone, and the next minute his face had smashed into the rear window of a stationary van. He was transferred to St George's by HEMS (helicopter emergency medical service). Multiple fractures had been wired and repaired during an eight-hour overnight operation. Skin had been removed from his upper arm and grafted onto his face.

This patient was in his mid-thirties. His face was very badly swollen. I switched off his sedation to wake him up, and the plan was to then extubate him (remove the breathing tube). In these situations, when a patient starts to wake, it's important to have a nurse there. I checked it was safe to remove the tube and, once he was fully awake, I ensured that he understood where he was and I explained the procedure so he could breathe normally.

When he was breathing normally, I started recording his observations. I wanted to count his respiratory rate but none of the clocks worked, so I couldn't see the time. We have all the high-tech monitors but, for an old-fashioned nurse, all that is needed to accurately count a respiratory rate is a clock with a second hand. I repeatedly glanced up at the clock on the wall above my bed space, which was stuck at 3.40. Each time I glanced I forgot that it would not be able to reveal the actual time, but still I

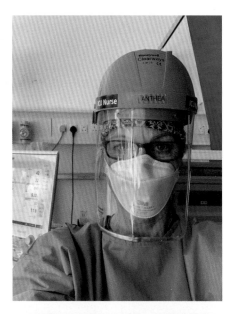

→ Brodie Ward,
April 2020

↓ Emma Dodi rainbow
cakes

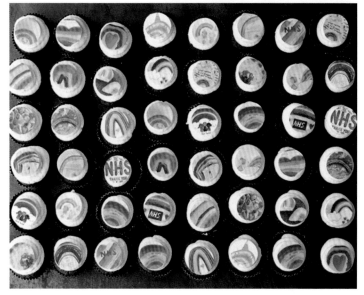

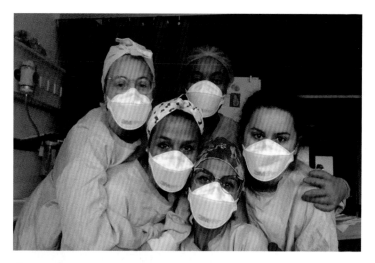

↑ Hugs, death and biscuits – European loving on Ben Weir Ward night shift

↓ The CriticalNhs food delivery crew

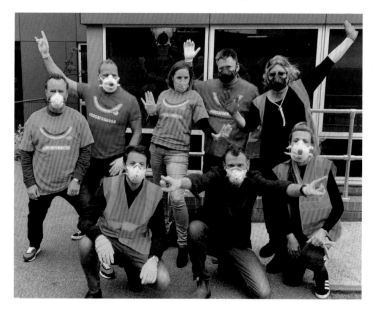

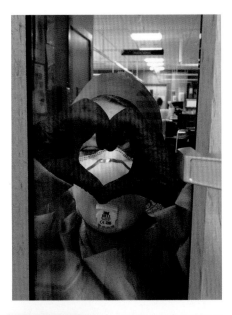

→ Melissa Walton – our very own Critical Care cover girl

↓ End-of-life compassion

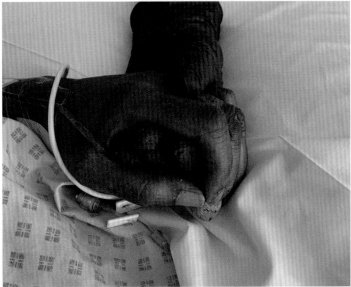

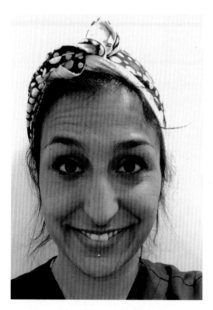

← Ilaria – night-duty face, London Scrubbers cap on

↓ European awesomeness – Ilaria and Monica

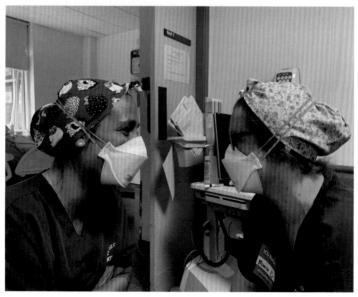

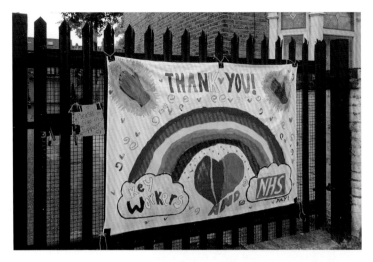

↑ A sign of gratitude to NHS and essential workers, London, May 2020

↓ Thursday clap from the St George's helipad, May 2020

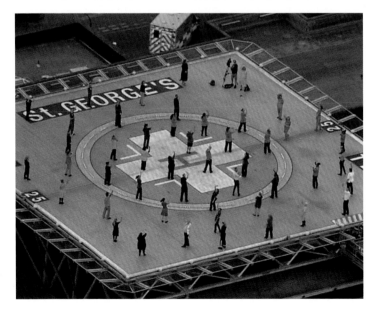

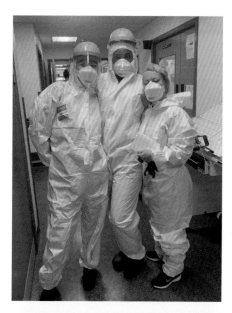

← Hazmat brigade

↓ Me and my Italian
and Portuguese
surrogate daughters

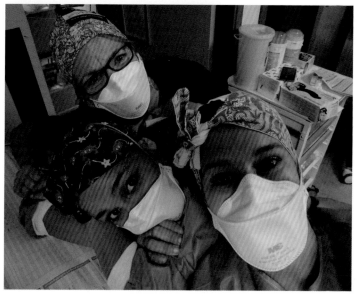

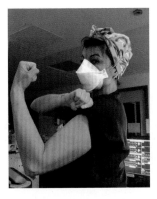

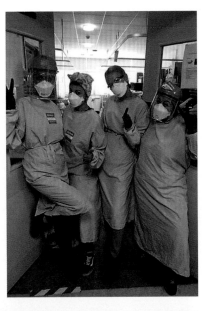

↑ Beatrice: 'We can do it!'

→ Girl power – Agnese, Beatrice, Laura and Alida

↓ Filipino-loving general ICU – Mary, Jessa and Justine

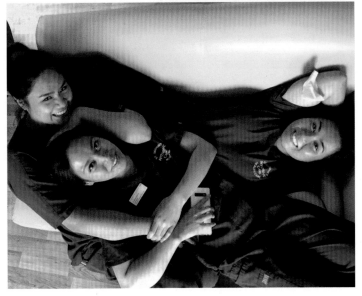

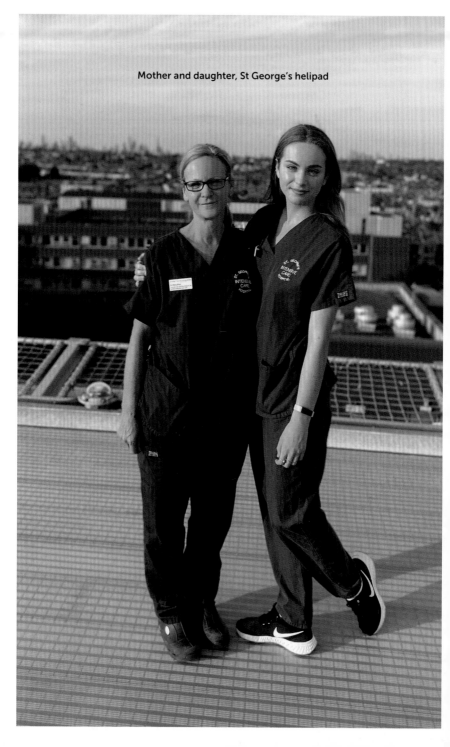

Mother and daughter, St George's helipad

kept looking at the broken clock. I said, 'Why are there no bloody batteries in the clock?' We are a centre of excellence but we always run out of AA batteries for the clocks. I made a fuss about this on numerous occasions throughout the day, and asked the technician and ward clerk to try to track down AA batteries. Six clocks were out of action due to dead batteries, which I found frustrating and ridiculous.

I am very tactile with the patients (we have to wear gloves), and I took his hand to connect with him and ensure he could understand what I was saying. It is important that a patient feels safe.

First thing in the morning, before he was extubated, he kept squeezing my arm and pulling it. I said, 'Can you hear me?' He nodded his head.

'Are you in pain?' I asked. He shook his head.

I said, 'You had an accident. Can you shut your eyes for me?' I wanted to check he was understanding me. He closed his eyes, and still he squeezed my hand and then rubbed it. He was anxious, and I could see his heart rate was 130 beats per minute on the monitor. I tried to calm him and get really good eye contact with him. Then my phone pinged with a WhatsApp message. He pointed at my phone.

I said, 'My phone? You want a phone? But you wouldn't be able to speak on the phone.' He kept pointing and trying to use his hand to gesticulate. I said, 'Buttons? Press buttons? You want to write something?' We continued like this, with me asking questions and him nodding or shaking his head.

Eventually, I said, 'Do you want to send an email?' Yes. 'So you want me to send an email. You need to send an email. This is an important email and if you don't send it there's a problem? OK, we can do this. And I'll do it on my phone. Who's the email to?'

He indicated to himself. 'Your whole name?' Yes. 'At Hotmail? At Google? Yahoo?' Through this strange, slow process I established his email address, and then that he wanted me to send a photograph of himself to his own email address. 'Do you know what you look like?' I said. 'You look really bad …' We were certainly communicating, even if it was taking a while.

Finally, under his instructions, I emailed a photograph of his face to himself, along with a message: 'I have had an accident and I am in St George's Hospital.'

'Sent,' I said. He settled down and went to sleep. Phew. That was exhausting. I told a few people about it. It was bizarre. His wife then arrived to visit. I told her about the email. She said, 'He works for a tech company and he's been organising this massive conference, and it starts this afternoon. Now that you've emailed his secretary, she will pick it up, see he's in hospital and understand. He's a very emotional, anxious person.' She sat by the bed while he slept.

Meanwhile, I was still grumbling about the clock that didn't work. Although he couldn't speak because his jaw was wired. His wife was holding the phone and they were sort of communicating with written messages that he typed with one finger, as his other arm was strapped up following the surgery to remove skin to transfer it onto his face.

When he was assessed and deemed fit enough to leave the ICU, I put him in a wheelchair and took him up to the ward. He kept stroking my arm.

His wife left and returned. She was holding a big bag. She said, 'I don't know what he's on about – and maybe he's a bit confused – but he asked me to go and buy this for you.' She handed me the bag. It was heavy and I thought, *That's a big box of chocolates.* Instead, the bag contained boxes of AA batteries – enough to keep the clock ticking for years and years. 'This,' I said to her, 'is the best present I've ever had.'

I put batteries in the clock, bringing it back to life, and then I asked one of the ward clerks to put new batteries in every single clock.

*   *   *

We continue the PPE theatrics at work and at home. No more than a group of six, unless you are being educated or exercising. We can spend the day together at work in a closed environment, with seven of us 'log rolling' a patient (turning an unconscious patient with a traumatic spinal cord injury while keeping the spine in alignment to prevent further injury). We are a few inches from one another, arms touching. But we cannot go out to dinner together – well, six of us can! I have a temperature check before my Pilates class or going onto a beach, but not before I enter the hospital.

A friend's daughter's best friend was in an accident. I can smuggle in a coffee from Pret and some chocolate, and pop by to say hello and give her a hug. For the staff, the strict rules around visitors are refreshing, though it must be so hard for the patients and the family who can only see loved ones via FaceTime or talk on the phone. I realise now how stressful relatives can be for the nurses, but it's understandable under the circumstances.

This girl is 18 years old and needs her family to visit. The physiotherapist, occupational therapist and nurses are her family for now, and me in my Mama Anthea role. I don't know this sparky, impressive young woman, but within seconds of meeting, the nurse-patient relationship kicks in and we are chatting like we have been close for years.

It's interesting and inspiring to still be learning about Critical Care and myself, even while heading towards retirement, which, incidentally, will never happen. Like my running, I will keep going until I can't keep going anymore.

We had a huge delivery of cake this week. A family dropped off homemade lemon drizzle and carrot cake. There was a card. It simply read, 'Thank you. You made such a difference.' If we can make a difference and in the future people look back and remember they had the best care and that we were kind – well, then we need no other appreciation (a pay rise, however, would be great).

Patients come and go. There is sadness, excellence, hilarity and celebration. We work hard. It's exhausting and can be unrelenting at times. During quieter periods, we wait for something to happen. Sometimes the individual we care for in the afternoon has just been living their life in the morning and has no idea that in a few hours they will be our patient. All the years I have worked on Critical Care, no day is anything like any other.

Running out of oxygen was a concern during Covid. Not enough staff or equipment or space. We discuss how we will deal with another surge. Will we learn from our last experience? It's like waiting for a bomb to explode.

We have been asked who will volunteer to go back. There is no choice, as far as I am concerned. It's like watching your home burn down. You sit and watch or help put out the fire. It's not a choice. What Critical Care nurses did during the pandemic is unmeasurable.

Many things have taken me back this week.

27 September

Claudia witnessed a cardiac arrest shortly after she started working with me. By the time she left, she had seen this happen on numerous occasions. Slick, structured, no-panic resuscitation. We have the equipment, staff and know-how, but still the sight is a shock to non-clinical staff.

A patient was so agitated, delirious and confused – as well as being young, tall and strong – that he was difficult to manage. There were a couple of occasions when he legged it down the corridor, with doctors and nurses in hot pursuit calling out instructions to obtain chemical restraint. This was given by intra-muscular injection in the lift lobby. The patient flopped gently to the floor, supported by staff, and was then carried back to bed.

This happened several times, our gently manhandling him in the corridor (on one occasion he was naked). This man was a danger to himself: drips and catheters yanked out, leaking a trail of blood behind him; without the oxygen he so needed. Unsafe.

The best way of caring for him was to put foam mattresses on the floor to stop him falling out of bed, and having an extra nurse sit by him at all times to maintain his safety and dignity. We jammed seven mattresses together in a secluded corner of Critical Care. He slept for hours, exhausted and recovering. We don't usually nurse people in this way, but he was safe.

It was an incredible day when he returned to visit. Sane, polite, well-dressed and nothing like the person he had been when recreational drugs had overwhelmed him. He had no idea about his frequent sprints along the corridor and out of Critical Care.

We prepare to surge. There is a tension in the hospital air. The numbers affected increase and we need to be able to hit the ground running. Once we start admitting people to Critical Care we will take transfers from 'out of area'. The waiting is harder than the doing, and we won't have enough trained staff.

I attended a meeting today. There were seven of us. One had to leave and attend via Microsoft Teams. I offered, but by the time I got back to my office and logged in, the meeting was over.

Organ donation continues. It's a tragedy when there is nothing left to do for an individual because their brain has died. The ventilator breathes for them and their heart contin-ues to pump oxygen around the body. But the person – the essence of who they are – has gone.

The most impossible and important decision a family can make is to donate their loved one's organs. Even if the patient is on the organ donor register it's a tough call. Our senior team for organ transplantation is incredible, and support and care and answer every question. It is so hard to accept that the person you love is brain dead when their chest moves up and down and their body is warm. A mum said to me once, 'My daughter died but her heart is still beating. And that gives me strength and courage each day.' Her daughter's heart is now owned by someone else.

I handed an elderly gentleman a cardboard urine bottle the other day. 'I can't piss in that!' he said. He couldn't walk to the toilet so there was little choice, and we had removed his cath-eter to progress his care and reduce the chance of him having an infection. Every piece of plastic we place in a person's body is a potential source of sepsis. So he had a wee on the floor before I was able to negotiate an alternative plan. The same shift a young woman vomited bile all over the wall and floor. My expertise was mostly employed that day with a mop.

The new junior doctors have started. I must be old, as they look so young and naive, but they are also keen and friendly. Fresh-faced and born in the mid-nineties, they have no actual idea of what they will see, learn or do. If they survive us, they will have completed their induction into medicine.

The team of Critical Care staff remains healthy. Through exposure perhaps we have gained a herd immunity. The toughest challenge would have been to nurse one of our own staff.

Covid updates are concerning and confusing. Perspective is often lost. Swirling insanity. Pubs closing early. 'Locktober' threatens us. The economy is collapsing. The environment polluted with masks. No one really knows how we should behave to maintain safety and prevent spreading the virus. So far it seems nothing has really made a difference. The weirdest rules are made about behaviour, and mask etiquette differs from one venue to another. Just know: if you come to hospital diagnosed with Covid-19, we will do the best we can. For now we have no Covid patients on Critical Care.

Electric scooters keep us busy: no helmet required and they can go fast. Swerving to avoid a cat and then flying into a brick wall can cause numerous facial fractures. A wired jaw means drinking fluids through a straw for weeks on end.

Sadly, this month we have lost four Spanish nurses, two Portuguese nurses, one Italian, a Greek nurse and one nurse from South America. All highly skilled, qualified and experienced Critical Care nurses, trained at St George's. They are delightful young people who have returned to their home country. Nursing in London is unsustainable. Low salary, high living cost, Brexit, and then there was Covid ...

Meanwhile, one nurse says to me, 'I wouldn't change the job I am in now. I would take the long hours, dehydration, weeing once in 13 hours – I'd take it all in return for the job satisfaction.'

OCTOBER 2020

4 October

In Britain, St George's is a lead site for one of the world's first phase 3 Covid-19 vaccine trials. The study will test the effectiveness of a new vaccine developed by Novavax. Whether or not there is a second wave, it seems that Covid is here to stay and we need to adapt our lives.

We have reason to be more confident this time. Our Covid Surge Critical Care area remains empty. I will be one of the senior staff who will board the spaceship if required. I am ready to don the dreaded PPE, permanently trying to avoid my glasses steaming up, ensuring a tight seal of my mask, which marks the face and makes the nose run. I remember taking a photo of a group of junior nurses in PPE, and one of them said, 'If only you could see the snot running down my face ...' We laughed – nurses often display dark and sardonic humour. We know no boundaries when it comes to discussing bodily fluids.

I transferred a patient to IR (Interventional Radiology) for a procedure that required X-ray imaging. Transporting a ventilated and unstable patient in a lift and then down the same corridor that leads to Pret is like being at the scene of an accident: people stop to watch while they are clutching their Americano, coconut latte or tea with almond milk (the variations on offer in coffee shops is remarkable).

This young woman, with four members of medical staff and two porters, looked so exposed and vulnerable, attached to a plethora of tubes and wires. I felt protective of her and uncomfortable that people would stare without shame. We are in a bubble in Critical Care; no one sees what happens or how people look. Transferring someone can destabilise them, and every nurse groans when they need to collect the kit required to transfer a patient for a procedure. Wires tangle, pumps alarm and the chaos created takes ages to unravel. We are not happy until our patient is pristine, untangled and back safely in their bed space 'owned' by the nurse of that shift. We are territorial of our space and protect our patient. It's usually one nurse to one level 3 patient, except during a pandemic when it changes drastically to an impossible patient–staff ratio.

One nurse was punched in the face by a confused patient. Her glasses broke. She took a moment, had a cup of tea and then went back to care for the man, mindful to duck his punches in future. Possibly he would never usually behave in such a way.

Experience is massive, and I have 24 years of it in Critical Care. I have a sixth sense. A 30 weeks pregnant woman required an emergency appendicitis and the obstetricians and surgeons worked together to perform the surgery. The obstetrician supported her enlarged uterus while the surgeon removed her appendix.

When I came on duty the next day the young mum was wandering around her bed, messaging her husband and small daughter. She was looking well but tired. She told me that the beds were so uncomfortable and that her back ached. She was fit to be discharged to a surgical ward. I saw her wince with pain and I put my hand on her tummy, which felt hard. I asked if she could be in labour and she said, 'I've had a baby before. This isn't what labour felt like.' I had a funny feeling and, despite there being a bed ready on a surgical ward, I refused to discharge her – to the annoyance of the consultant and matron. I was in charge; this was my shift and I stood by my gut instinct – something wasn't right. A compromise was made and later in the day she was transferred to a labour ward to be observed overnight, and then she would be transferred to a surgical ward in the morning.

Late that evening I received a text message from a colleague. The patient had delivered her premature baby five minutes after arriving on the labour ward. The appropriate staff were available and the baby boy was transferred to the neonatal unit. He was discharged home, fit and well, six weeks later.

I always trust my instincts.

My European nurses teach me a range of words and sentences in their own language and then roar with laughter at my mispronunciation. This works both ways. I permanently adopt some of their sentences as we do with children who mispronounce a word that becomes forevermore a family word. An Italian nurse suggested we order a 'Thailandish' takeaway. Thai food to me now is always Thailandish.

* * *

As the weather changes we are starting to see chest infections, seasonal illnesses that deteriorate with the weather, chronic respiratory issues requiring support. We have a few people with lungs that are non-compliant and failing. If these patients are ventilated they will never be able to breathe unaided. Some require non-invasive ventilation, when a fitted mask is required to help expand their lungs. Claustrophobic and tight, I have heard patients say.

Sometimes we need to have a conversation to discuss this, and it's complex if the patient does not agree with their family. A man said to his wife, 'Come on, love. I smoked all my life. I knew the risks. I don't want a machine to breathe for me. It's time to go ...' So hard, but the patient made his own decision. The following evening he died, in comfort with his wife by his side.

I have mentioned the doors before. Often broken or stiff, or on a go-slow with the right-hand door flying open and beds and trolleys crashing against the left-hand one slowly opening. The double doors to the staff corridor are stiff. I can spot our regular staff – you press the green button on the wall, then whack your right hip against the right-hand door and they open. Critical Care non-residents press the button and gently push – nothing happens.

If the doors were ever fixed, we would see countless staff go through the motions with the green button, a swing of their hip, only to fall through the door as it opened with ease like a normal door.

So no surge yet. Each week that I write, I wonder if next week will be different and the tsunami will hit. Last time it seemed to change overnight. The rage train took us by surprise. Not this time. We are ready. Let's see.

We wait. We had no idea how long it would last for, but we expected that one wave of the virus would be replaced months later by another. I work in a brilliant hospital, and if you come here sick or injured, there's a very strong chance that you will receive exceptional care and kindness, and will recover. How long does it take to get better? I am not sure, but be prepared to wait in order to be well. In hospitals you'll hear medical staff tell a patient, 'We'll come and get you at ten.' I never say that sort of thing because it means the patient is waiting for ten o'clock, at which point nothing happens, no one comes.

Instead, I say, 'When I was in Malaysia, I was getting a boat, and I asked when it was coming. They said, "In between now and a little while …" That is how long it takes.' Patients understand that. That's an NHS ten minutes

Happy Sunday everyone. I am just off to run a half-marathon in the pouring rain.

10 October

An elderly woman had chronic obstructive pulmonary disease (COPD), which causes long-term breathing problems. She was recovering from a chest infection and receiving oxygen via nasal cannula. She asked if I could find her handbag. I found it in the trolley by her bed and handed it to her. She rummaged around in the detritus within her bag. She produced many tissues, a lipstick, a notebook, pen, purse, hairbrush, umbrella, travel card, as well as various items you would expect to find in an elderly lady's handbag.

I was talking to another nurse a few metres away. I glanced up after a few moments to see a cigarette between the patient's lips. She sparked the disposable lighter and took an enormous drag on her freshly lit fag. I was a bit shocked. Was I seeing correctly? She took one more puff. I launched forward and grabbed the impending fire risk away from her mouth and the flow of oxygen around her nose. She was slightly disgruntled but easily distracted with a cup of tea.

I have had Instagram tutorials from the juniors, who never get frustrated by my clumsy screen tapping and swiping, searching for the correct emoji or boomerang. The medical abbreviation for fracture is #, now universally known as the hashtag sign on social media. Some of us older ones had a hilarious moment when a junior doctor asked what a 'hashtag hip' was.

Well, it isn't happening, this global disease that is casting a shadow across the world. We wait to enter our bio bubble, but not quite yet. I remember before, when we were waiting, preparing our surge areas that admitted more and more patients. Senior staff from the three Critical Care areas would meet daily in the morning on cardiac ICU to discuss appropriate staffing levels, discharges, admissions and transfers, so that we knew our bed capacity for emergency and elective admissions. Suddenly, there were seven areas, with more and more staff. We had to relocate our meeting. Elective surgery was cancelled and we would just keep admitting Covid patients. A person would die and then another would arrive, and another and another ... It was frightening. The anticipation became a reality and tension filled the air.

We didn't know how to manage it. We just had to make the best plan we could as a team and try to keep up with the pace – Covid positive patients were being admitted at alarming rates. We were frightened. My heart rate increases just remembering that time, and I understand why such bonds were formed.

A man was admitted via our Emergency Department (ED), inebriated and waiting to go to theatre. He had been found by the police, wandering along the train tracks looking for his dog – he didn't own a dog. He was badly injured when he was presumably hit by a train. He didn't remember. He needed to go to theatre to have his injuries cleaned and repaired. No dog was found on the tracks.

The technical equipment we use can be mind-blowing. So many modes, variations and buttons to manipulate precisely an amount of drug, blood or air required by our ventilators, filters and pumps. These machines are frequently upgraded to the latest model with yet more bells and whistles and flashing lights. When I first started working in Critical Care, I would hear the alarm sounds of the machines in my sleep: each has its own unique ear-piercing or monotonous alarm. I tell patients' loved ones that they act as alarm clocks to remind nurses of a required impending action, rather than always screeching out an emergency. It's like being on a plane during turbulence: the seat belt sign goes on and we glance at the cabin crew; if they are calm and carry on, we know all is fine. It's the same in Critical Care. Some visitors jump out of their skin when a monitor or pump alarms. If the nurses act calmly then there is no emergency.

Breaking bad news is hard. Some staff handle it better than others. No matter how senior a member of staff is, it is a challenging situation. No amount of training can help – it's instinct and compassion that are important. We need to be clear and unambiguous, and use words a family will understand. Euphemisms are unhelpful. We talk about the 'D' word. If a person is going to die then a family needs to know this. 'Passed on' or 'passed away' or 'go to the little place in the sky' are unclear. Family need to know, understand and then accept the inevitable. It's by far the best way if we are kind and clear and answer all questions.

Years ago a junior nurse called a family to tell them that their loved one was fit for discharge to the ward. They were on their way to visit. A sudden and unexpected collapse by the patient resulted in CPR being in progress when they arrived.

The family were asked by the receptionist to wait. After some time, and once the gentleman was pronounced dead, the junior nurse went to see the family, and said that a doctor was on their way to update them. His wife wanted immediate detail so the nurse gently explained that he had collapsed and staff had tried to resuscitate him, and the wife was gently informed that he had 'passed on'.

'Thank God for that,' she said. 'For a moment there I thought you were telling me he had died. Which ward did he pass on to?'

Death and dying are a natural part of life, but these words make many people feel uncomfortable or anxious. Passed on, deceased, didn't make it, snuffed it, kicked the bucket, gave up the ghost, slipped away, breathed their last breath, lost the battle, curtains – so many ways to say one word. Helpful or harmful? It's important to be clear. Death is final and that word is final. It communicates absolutely that a person has died and therefore their life has been extinguished.

I have learned over the years to be direct and not skirt around the issue. Words and phrases like brain dead, suicide and unsurvivable are hard to hear. And it never becomes any easier for the member of staff communicating this shocking and devastating news. I have trained myself not to cry – it's not my grief, but it doesn't mean we don't identify with the situation. My heart goes out to families and loved ones. We never 'harden'; we just learn to manage our own feelings. It makes me sad if someone says nurses 'harden', because we don't at all. If we become hard it's time to stop and find an alternative career.

*   *   *

ICU nurses really know and appreciate the value of personal care. At the height of the tsunami it was almost impossible to give patients the care they would usually receive. I was with two young nurses as they discussed their highs of the pandemic.

First young nurse: 'One of the best feelings that I had in Brodie was the first time I could shave a patient. I felt so happy the first time I saw my patient without a beard.'

Second young nurse: 'I remember I was on Brodie, and the sun was coming up. It was a night shift, no one had died and it was a really lovely sunny morning, and I had brushed a patient's teeth. And I was like, *Wow, what a good day.*'

18 October

A patient was dying. In her eighties, she had been ill for some time. Her two daughters were with her, the curtains drawn together around the bed to give the illusion of privacy. My colleague could hear their voices, at first muted but gradually the volume increased. They were arguing about their mum's belongings. The main area of dispute seemed to be her jewellery. It appeared they agreed on very little, actually. Eventually, they became so loud they had to be asked to be a bit quieter. It was suggested that they use the time they had to talk to their mum and say goodbye. A little part of me hopes the patient has left her jewellery to somebody else.

A woman in her eighties, who has lived alone since her husband's death over 10 years ago, has two daughters who visit regularly and several grandchildren. She was independent, fit and healthy. Loved visiting National Trust properties with her best friend and was known for her jam-making skills. She drove her own car and had no significant health problems.

During a trip to the supermarket, a fellow shopper accidentally caught her ankle with their shopping trolley. A bruise developed into a haematoma (a blood collection under the surface of the skin). This required surgical removal, as it was causing pressure within her leg. The wound became septic and she required multiple trips to theatre to have her leg cleaned and debrided (cleaning a wound and removing dead skin and tissue).

She required intravenous antibiotics and developed a hospital-acquired pneumonia (HAP). When her wound healed, she would require reconstructive plastic surgery. This elderly patient lost her appetite and required a nasogastric tube to be fed. She didn't even have the appetite to try the homemade soup made by her granddaughter.

Her limbs developed generalised oedema (fluid collection within the tissue), which also affected the healing of her wound.

She became delirious and agitated, and pulled out her drips and repeatedly removed the high-flow oxygen administered by nasal cannula, causing her oxygen levels to drop. We sedated her and I held her hand as the anaesthetist intubated her.

This was an accident, but the elderly seem to tip so quickly. From independence to total dependence, thus hugely increasing her chance of mortality. The likelihood of this lovely woman returning to her pre-accident health and quality of life were fast diminishing. Had this happened to a teenager, there would probably be a bruise, some hopping and bad language, and they would most likely heal.

Health deteriorates with age, as does our ability to heal and recover. The body's resilience is not as good as it once was. She did recover but her foot was finally amputated and she was discharged to the ward. I have no idea what happened after that. When a patient leaves ICU we rarely discover what happens in the end.

The fellow shopper will not know any of this. It was an accident, and accidents can, in a second, change a person's life irrevocably.

*　　*　　*

The guys have set up a group to play a weekly football match and, to counterbalance it, the girls have started a netball team. One of our practice educators (clinical teachers) was limping around the unit the day after a match, during which he had bruised muscles he never knew he had. It's great to see the staff play sport together, and they are pretty fit and competitive, having infiltrated each other's teams and having even recruited the rep for our new haemofiltration machines, who has joined in to score a few goals and is particularly impressive at netball. I have seen some astonishing bruises. We are brilliant at teamwork and it translates well onto the pitch.

Pre-Covid, a woman was very sick after a spontaneous and massive bleed in her brain – a subarachnoid haemorrhage. She sang in a gospel choir, and her daughter asked if some members of the choir could come in and sing for her unconscious mum. We had a fabulous Friday evening when five singers from this lady's church sang their hearts out at her bedside, filling Critical Care with song. So uplifting and beautiful.

The patient made a full recovery, against all odds. She puts it down to the excellent care she received. I like to think the singing had something to do with it.

We are back to wearing FFP3 masks. Our devices manager says they smell of caraway, but to me they smell of Covid and they propel me back to a place I can't explain. A few nurses found it tough putting the masks back on – it catapults us to hell. One nurse had a panic attack and was so upset that she needed to go home.

Suppressing the fear factor is exhausting. We are mostly busy but Covid took busy to another level and we remain bruised. I still reflect on specific situations and wonder if I could have done something differently. Could we have done more, or done it better? Frequently we felt guilty. I felt guilty when I wasn't at work, which was why I would often go in on my day off. I needed to be there. We were paid for the extra days we worked.

There are now five Covid-positive patients requiring Critical Care. Once we reach six patients it is our trigger to escalate and recreate a Covid ICU on the ward where we were before. This means decanting 28 non-Covid surgical cardiac patients to other areas and discharging the fit patients home. Not a mean feat, relocating so many patients. We will then clean the area and set it up yet again, creating Critical Care space in a non-Critical Care environment.

There are dozens of ventilators covered in plastic at the back of the staff canteen. It's like eating lunch at a sci-fi convention, with little aliens waiting for action. In the first surge it was mind blowing – all the different ventilators, and each patient seemed to be attached to a different model. If we surge again, our Head of Clinical Engineering says that the Covid areas will have all the same make and model of ventilators, pumps and monitors as far as possible.

Previously we set up a Stab Room – a stabilisation room where a patient is intubated (breathing tube inserted), and an arterial line, CVC (central venous catheter), peripheral cannulas (drips) and nasogastric tube (for feeding or drainage) are inserted. These lines and tubes are essential for taking blood to analyse oxygenation and blood chemistry, for feeding a patient, and they are required for drug administration via a pump. Some drugs called inotropes, which support cardiac function, are calculated at micrograms per kilogram per minute – precise amounts.

Sedation, analgesia, antibiotics, antivirals, steroids, blood products, fluids and other life-saving medication are also given via infusion, thus requiring a bank of pumps and syringe drivers stacked on a drip pole next to the bed. We also insert a urinary catheter to measure and analyse urine. Some patients require chest tubes to drain blood or fluid from the lungs, and a large cannula in the neck or groin for filtration or dialysis.

Once stabilised, the patient is moved safely to a permanent bed space. Sometimes we are not able to stabilise these patients and that is when they die.

The kit required for our surge area will be taken and set up in preparation for the storm. We then lock it down for Covid and board the express train.

At the moment there are only five patients. One admission, one death or one recovery could change everything. If we need to open, it will happen fast and meticulously. Our staff will step up and be brilliant. We have the hand of history on our shoulders. We can do more than we think we can.

'No human is limited,' said Eliud Kipchoge. One of my heroes, who in 2019 became the first person to run the marathon distance of 26.2 miles in under two hours.

20 October

Jonathan Silver, the Head of Clinical Engineering (as well as making great sourdough) has returned to Facebook. On the subject of ventilators he writes, 'We have more than twice as many as we had in March ... Only about half of them are "top of the range" and are what we might consider buying ourselves; the rest of them are "last season" – released in 2003, or the slightly more basic model intended for developing markets instead of western Europe – but they are all good machines and will allow us to provide the care we need to. It's a bit disheartening that we are now (gratefully) accepting ventilators of the type we gave away a few years ago because we'd upgraded to a later model. But, sadly, squirrelling old equipment away for once-in-a-lifetime pandemics never featured on our radar, or any national guidance ...

'As the Covid patients piled in during March and April, the rest of the hospital was fairly quiet. The overall number of unplanned admissions plunged. Many people were too scared to come to hospital when they were unwell ... Tragically, we suspect many people may have suffered and died at home, in spite of our pleas on social media to come in if they needed treatment. Our usually packed medical wards ended up half empty, and only just in time – we needed every spare nurse to support the onslaught in the temporary ICUs ... And the number of planned admissions plunged as well ... Besides, our anaesthetists and vital equipment were all borrowed from theatres and were needed in intensive care.

'This time, as the numbers increase, the aspiration is to continue with everything: scan everyone, treat everyone, keep all theatres open. The government are pushing this very hard.' And, particularly now that it's winter and everyone's bored with the pandemic, I don't think we'll see people shying away from coming to ask for help when they need it. And so, instead of starting the onslaught with a third of our beds empty, we're already full to bursting. We coped last time because we had the space to, but this time it will be a very different challenge.'

26 October

I don't even know how to begin.

Last weekend five patients became three, so the Covid Express train remained at the station. Every day we wondered what to expect. We stood at the edge of the cliff, ready to fall. Then, on Tuesday, three became four, then five and then seven. And today we have nine patients. The most recent patient needed to be proned, so here we go again ...

It feels like we are in reverse at 70 mph. It's so weird, like being on one of those rollercoasters at a theme park that you want to get off as soon as it starts to climb the initial upward section of the track.

It's exactly the same as before. We can't breathe, and most nurses have only just begun to recover from last time – if at all. There is an entire army of fantastic people who make the day to day happen, but I am a nurse and it's the

Critical Care nurses in particular who take the unrelenting brunt of it.

Last night, the clocks went back an hour, so nurses spent almost 14 hours working in our recently set up Covid area. Some of them didn't want to go back, but they are nurses; there is no choice. Our brains are rushing to process this reality, using the frame of reference we built the last time it happened. Do we really have to do this again? Can we? We thought it would happen but mentally it's difficult to prepare for something that may happen and that we dread.

Our systems and methods, how we stored fluid, where we kept ventilator tubing, where the extra oxygen cylinders were kept – we have to rebuild, recreate and start all over again. The windows closed, the air-con off, PPE suffocating us. The hospital has already emailed Claudia and asked her to come back. She is back at uni now, so she can't.

We have already moved away from the imagery, the demons, the fear, and now we need to step over the threshold again. The difference now is that we know how it is and how it will be. We are scared. I am scared for myself and for those young, beautiful nurses who now have a place in my heart. We ask nurses to do this for nothing, no reward, no bonus, no pay rise, no extra day off, no free coffee, and please don't clap this time. We know it's our job, but it isn't really. THIS IS BEYOND, but we carry on regardless.

We tip at a restaurant, even if the service is not great – 10 per cent added to the bill. Nurses get nothing yet do so much, and I only give you a glimpse of the reality.

It's odd when home and work collide. I remember seeing one of Claudia's teachers in Critical Care when she was visiting her father. It was so weird: one minute discussing Claudia's homework, the next her father's imminent death. We both had to find a professional balance.

I nursed someone in my Pilates class, though she did not make the connection and I haven't reminded her. But the strangest time involved a young man who had been knocked off his bike by a truck and was recovering well following pelvic surgery. When I helped him put a T-shirt on, I noticed that it was the same finisher top that I'd also received after completing a half-marathon a few weeks earlier. I fell during the race but was scooped up by two runners who came to my rescue. I caught my breath, hobbled a bit and was then fine to keep running and finish the 12.1-mile race.

I said I had run the same race. He told me he'd been aiming for a fast time to secure a place in the London Marathon, which was now irrelevant due to his bike accident. 'It was a great race,' he said, 'until some bird tripped over in front of me, so me and my mate stopped to help her.'

'That was me!' We had such a laugh together, and what a coincidence.

We are aiming to keep normal services up and running. To keep admitting patients following accident, illness, injury and essential surgery. Each day, staff are allocated to a particular area. I am senior but I don't know where I will work on Wednesday – Covid DIY, Critical Care or 'home' on my own unit in a different wing of the hospital. This is the NHS, and even though we have done it before, it doesn't mean we are set up, prepared and ready for action. Saving money is important, so a decision is made last minute and then it's all systems go, which adds to chaos and anxiety.

We have new junior doctors; some are fresh out of medical school. It's particularly tough for our new staff and for those relocated to help, with no preparation or warning. Student nurses and retired nurses whose registration have lapsed come to help, some by choice, some not, defying their expectations of themselves. They have no script; they have just landed in this apocalyptic upheaval. We have a symbiotic relationship with Covid. We fight it, we work with it, we defend our patients. I find it odd that so few of us have been grasped by the tentacles of Covid and succumbed to it.

So floral cloth hats back on, we march forward, towards the enemy, and my peripheral vision keeps an eye on my fabulous colleagues. Sense of humour intact, we start all over again.

NOVEMBER 2020

1 November

Our makeshift Critical Care spaceship is up and running. It's like stepping back in time. I am in charge today. My first shift back at the helm since we closed in July. Some of the incredible support team have popped up again, ward staff, uni students and ex-ICU nurses. This time we have the army to help too.

The patients are all Covid-positive. Some are improving and some deteriorating. An elderly man, an ex-pilot, said to me, 'The nurses here are so amazing it actually makes my heart ache. I am 81, alive and better. And I will make the very best of the time I have left. The positivity here is like medicine.'

The day is going fast, the team efficient and brilliant, making decisions about each individual patient and what we can do to help them improve. We discuss curative and supportive care. There is no definitive treatment, but we now know what may help: which drugs, which therapy and even which pressures to set on the ventilator. We give steroids to reduce pulmonary inflammation, anticoagulant to reduce the chance of a blood clot, and anti-viral therapies, while frequently needing to paralyse and sedate patients (induced medical coma) to manage their respiratory failure. We deliver high-quality clinical care.

The medical team today are on fire: up to date on the latest Covid research, adjusting medication doses and interventions to maximise the best treatment; involving other specialists and taking time to do the best thing for each person. I am in awe of the expertise and knowledge. We work as a team. Input from everyone is valued and considered.

The Covid-19 pandemic led to an unprecedented surge in hospitalised patients with viral pneumonia, but we are learning how to treat this and when to stop. There is a threshold, and once a patient reaches this on the ward they are transferred to Critical Care so their worsening symptoms can be managed and supported in a timely manner.

Patients are scared, especially if they see others around them deteriorate or die and wonder if this is their trajectory. We do all we can to help them feel safe. Currently we have approximately 20 patients on the Covid ward and 11 patients on Covid ICU. But this changes day by day and sometimes hour by hour. Clinical trials continue to add to the body of knowledge.

The most severely affected patients were middle-aged men last time, often of black and Asian minority ethnicity, and those with comorbidities (pre-existing illness or ill health). This time, however, I am surprised by how many of our patients are women. Who knows how this virus chooses its pathway; perhaps this is just for this week.

One of our junior nurses is dealing with many issues at home. She has a parent with mental-health challenges, and I am in awe of her work ethic and attitude while also committed to supporting her parent.

Another nurse works all day and returns home to her husband with MND (motor neurone disease). She takes over from the carer at home, having been a carer all day herself. Another nurse returned for her first shift today after maternity leave. As she is working amidst the Covid patients she is concerned about her baby. And a Filipino nurse has been receiving messages from home about Typhoon Goni. She showed me a photo of her friend, waist high in water, whose home had already been destroyed.

We are invincible. We have a wicked sense of humour, sense of fun and excellent work ethic, as well as the ability to devour pizza in record time. We also show compassion and genuinely care about our patients.

It is weirdly OK to be back. I was apprehensive when my alarm went off at 5 a.m. this morning. We are used to the PPE and the way of working. There is a good team on duty. We have got the iPads up and running, navigating the poor Wi-Fi connection. I have changed the batteries in the clocks, restocked some cupboards and moved the bin to a better position. Our hero ward clerk stood on a chair to reposition a sign that was wonky. There were raptures when we fixed the label machine, and I am happy that the settings on the PC have been reconfigured to print out the patient list in the correct order. We are nesting, making this odd space our home.

The nurses work hard to keep to the daily routine while always being prepared for the unexpected. As the nurse in charge, I walk miles each day, in and out of the pods to give support, advice, reassurance, assistance or fetch and carry as required.

Lockdown is going to be harder this time. The weather has changed and people are bored and impatient. I gain so much from our team spirit, which is what keeps us all going. We are lucky, as we are immersed in people at work while others may be lonely and trapped at home. Lockdown may help defeat the virus but is this going to provoke a mental-health deterioration pandemic?

One of our Italian nurses is leaving to return home. The pandemic has highlighted her need to be with her family. When I left our Covid ICU this evening, after handing over to the nurse in charge of the night shift, I returned to my ICU to get changed and collect my bag. There were many tears, as she had just finished her last shift. Her friends were crying because she was going, and she was crying because she was leaving a job and colleagues she loves.

We are quite a soppy lot, really. Amidst the tears there were flowers, gifts and cards, homemade cake and the obligatory dips and carrot sticks from M&S.

She will keep in touch, but not if I ever eat pineapple on my pizza. It is an Italian law, I have learned, that this must never happen!

*   *   *

My mum worked in Casualty, as the Emergency Department was called then. She would often work night shifts. As I've mentioned, before I left for school each morning, I would sit on our front porch and wait for the car to come up the driveway. It meant I could grab a kiss and listen to her tell me stories about what had happened in her life while I'd slept.

I am known for my storytelling and I now know where this comes from. Just as I have done with my children, she would tell me stories in which the detail increased the older I became. Stories about her shift, the patients, the staff and the security guard's Alsatian dog who was soppy and unlikely to act as a guard dog in any situation – always preferring a tummy rub. She told stories of confused patients, missing dentures and the crazy that was – and still is – hospital life on the front line.

It was around this time that I knew I wanted to be a nurse. My mum's job sounded exciting and fun and amazing, but it was more than that. It wasn't a decision for me; it was something I needed to do, and still do. Looking back, I also realise I inherited the random parenting gene, directed at the younger nurses. When I first qualified, I worked Christmas morning and drove home after work to find three young women sitting by the Christmas tree, playing with our dog. My mum had also been working and these Irish nurses couldn't get home for Christmas, so she had invited them to share festive celebrations with us. We had a fantastic day. My parents seemed to unearth extra food and crackers. We ate, drank, played games and had such fun.

Every Boxing Day we'd pile into the car and drive over to my aunt's home, where we'd have lunch and exchange Christmas presents. One Boxing Day we were driving home and passed an accident. 'Let's pull over,' said my mother. She got out of the car and ran back to see what she could do, how she could help. I was in the back seat and turned around to peer through the rear window, desperate to catch a glimpse of the action. It was too dark for me to see what was happening, with only a mass of silhouettes visible against the headlights of the oncoming cars. But again, it was a moment of excitement. And again, I thought, 'I want to do that.'

Then there was that time when my parents threw a fancy-dress party, to which guests were invited to come as either a saint or a sinner. Our house was filled with lots of my mother's nurse and doctor friends – angels with wings, bishops in robes or priests in dog collars, devils and demons. During the party there was an accident on the road outside our home; two teenagers had been hit by a speeding car. My parents' guests instinctively rushed to help – in their fancy dress – and I watched in awe as my mother dressed the lads' injuries. One of the guests, who'd come to the party as a policeman, took full advantage of his costume by waving oncoming vehicles away from the scene of the accident.

The lads were taken to hospital, and when my mother went to work the next day she popped in to see how they were getting on. They were both doing well, but one of them recalled, 'I was lying there, surrounded by angels and men in robes ... I thought I was in heaven.'

One morning, when I was about nine, my mum returned home from her night shift crying. It had been snowing heavily and was icy cold outside, so I wasn't waiting on the porch. She walked into our kitchen and burst into tears. I don't think I had ever seen her cry and it unnerved me. My father hugged her tightly. She told us about the nurse in charge from the day shift who had handed over to my mum. The nurse had just returned from her honeymoon and showed my mum her wedding photos. Later that evening the ambulance crew brought in a patient. Cardiopulmonary resuscitation was being performed. They used to call this a 'suspended' patient, as if the patient were suspended between life and death. My mum said one of the team pulled a face at her, gesturing towards the patient and shaking his head.

Lying there was the same, just-married nurse who had handed over to my mum. She was now a patient with a tube in her throat, her colleagues performing CPR. Resuscitation was abandoned after one hour by medical staff who knew her and worked with her, doing all they could to ignite life back into her soul.

I don't remember the rest of the detail. Something about the gas boiler in the bathroom being blocked with snow, and her falling asleep in the bath while drinking a glass of wine. What I do remember is my mum's distress. And I remember her saying that losing a colleague is a strange feeling. Not really a friend or family, but someone you see often, someone you like and respect and are closely connected to, this relationship is never considered. I have since experienced this close bond with colleagues but never so much as during Covid times.

The relationship nurses have with one another is intimate and deep seated and unfathomable. Some of us become friends and some do not. Nevertheless, there is a bond derived from understanding, experience and something else that I cannot explain.

11 November

Today I received the most wonderful email from Dr Tim Evans. Dr Evans is Apothecary to Her Majesty the Queen and the Royal Households of London. He has been reading and enjoying my weekly messages from the front line. Imagine my reaction. Spirits mightily boosted and feeling terribly flattered, I can't help wondering if he shared any of my emails with the Queen.

*   *   *

'Still terrifying.' That is how Jonathan Silver describes the situation. 'But perhaps for different reasons this time,' he says. 'Sometimes the known is scarier than the unknown. Last time we had no idea what the challenge was going to be, and we knew we wouldn't get everything right and would need to learn as we went; now we have looked the beast in the face, the pressure feels very different.'

What makes it feel different, he adds, is that in March and April, the world stopped. There were no distractions, nothing else to do but focus on the task in hand. 'For five or six weeks I couldn't string a sentence together at home, but it didn't matter. Now, for better or worse, the world keeps spinning. There is still music making, there are friends and family to see (outside), the pubs are open (sort of). These are important and brilliant things. But they mean that, if everything goes south and the days grow long again, I can't afford to be so absorbed, and will have to start actually planning my time again – which is hard when your decision fatigue already sets in halfway through the working day.'

21 November

Some of our patients are obese. It takes at least three or four nurses to turn them and then reposition them to prevent pressure sores and to support respiratory function and improve oxygenation. Immobility is associated with complications, so it is important that we turn our patients every few hours. Last week one of the nurses brought a massage gun to work, and we took turns massaging each other's backs with this vibrating machine – so much hilarity. Our backs often ache after a shift of turning, rolling, bending, twisting, lifting. We have annual updates on how to safely move patients to protect us and them, using appropriate equipment. But some days it is relentless and we just ache.

A Covid-positive patient woke during the night. She said she had dreamed of eating poppyseed cake, which she frequently baked on her farm in Cornwall. And because, coincidentally, we had some poppyseed cake remaining from our weekly sweet treat delivery from a local friend, we were able to fulfil her dream. She devoured a huge slice of said cake at 3 a.m. and then went back to sleep. It's these little things that are the best of nursing.

Yesterday my patient was extremely unstable and it was a challenge to keep his blood pressure and ventilation appropriate for his needs. He was trying to die. We fix the problem if we can and treat the best way we can. At one point I counted 11 people around the bed space, doctors and nurses all there for the purpose of delivering the best possible treatment required. Re-intubation and ventilation; the insertion of a chest drain and a bronchoscope (a device used to see inside the airways and lungs); then an echocardiogram followed by an X-ray: he was fixed, and 100 per cent oxygen became 25 per cent by the end of my shift.

Arbitrary restrictions become so bizarre. Wandering around the supermarket, life is the same except for the masks, no one really paying attention to the arrow signs illustrating the direction you should walk in. No lockdown visible. I can be with my colleagues at work but not at their home. We are so physically close during some medical procedures but we cannot sit in groups of more than six in the coffee room. In some ways we are lucky. We are connected by an invisible bond that we all understand and recognise, and it will last a lifetime. There are so many of us. We can laugh and chat and be together, but I am aware that there are some lonely people out there, craving human contact, estranged from family and friends. Surely those with challenges to their mental health build resilience by contact with others. We may help defeat the virus, but at what cost?

Winking is suddenly important. If you see someone you know, you smile. Even if you don't know them, you might smile. With a mask they can't see you smile except from your eyes. If you want them to know you are smiling – you wink. I am lucky. I can wink with both eyes, and I now wink a lot! Much can be communicated with a wink.

Patients who test positive come to our dedicated area and we do what we can. It is still emotionally traumatic when a person dies but, although we have lost a few patients, it's not quite as before. We are skilled and experienced and ready. Every day more patients arrive, threatening to fill our Covid area. Plans are afoot to surge into a second area, but then one patient dies and another is discharged to the ward, and we have space.

It's been quite a process setting up and creating our makeshift ICU as it was last time. Everything had been packed up and stored, and we are aiming to mimic the same systems and stock the cupboards as before. I am still looking in the wrong place for items that are always needed in a hurry. And the support nurses look blankly at you when you ask them to find something they have never heard of. They learn to think on their feet and find an HME (Heat and Moisture Exchanger for the ventilator), syringes, an ECG (electrocardiogram) cable, a body bag, a specific dressing ... We shall get there.

We are a slightly changed team but it is not taking long to get back into the system we left in the summer. The PPE is familiar now and we know how to work while wearing it.

Spirits are fairly good. We are nurses. We have bounced back well. It's just exhausting sometimes and wounds have only just healed. Let's hope we don't have to do it for long this time.

> 'Be kind whenever possible.
> It's always possible.'
>
> *The Dalai Lama*

*   *   *

Nursing rotas are based on a 37.5-hour week. Though, of course, we work more hours than that. Our meal breaks are deducted, which makes no sense, as we frequently skip our breaks, especially during Covid times.

Many years ago, I owed four hours so I came into work mid-afternoon on a Friday to complete the time deficit. I had been qualified for one year and was working on a medical ward at St George's. My long-term plan was to work in Casualty, which was subsequently renamed Accident & Emergency (A&E) and more recently Emergency Department (ED). There is no difference but all the signage needs changing every time.

I like drama. Trauma, severe illness and injury are fascinating. I found the environment stimulating and exciting, and after an eight-week stint there as a student nurse, that was my plan – but plans change.

I arrived at work on this particular Friday and the nurse in charge asked me to collect a patient from the endoscopy unit, in another wing on the far side of the hospital, and bring them back to the ward.

When I arrived in Endoscopy the patient didn't look quite right; nothing specific, I just had a feeling. A quick look at his vital signs told me he wasn't adequately oxygenated, so I sat him upright on the trolley to improve his lung expansion, started oxygen and waited. He was only in his forties, and sleepy and breathless following his bronchoscopy (a procedure to look at the lungs and air passages). He slowly improved and, as 5 p.m. approached, there was pressure to leave, as the unit was closing for the day. My patient was the last patient and was now fit to leave for the ward.

I was a bit concerned but a porter arrived to push the trolley with me. The receptionist said she would walk with us to help, as I wanted to borrow some of the monitoring equipment. A locum anaesthetist asked for directions to the theatres in St James Wing, so I suggested he join the entourage and I would show him, as it was en route.

The transfer did not go to plan. My first experience of gut instinct as a nurse was correct. After jolting the trolley through the bowels of Knightsbridge Wing (a building since demolished), a ride in a lift, and then weaving our way via a glass link corridor, my patient suddenly looked dreadful. He became sweaty and quiet; his lips were blue and his eyes moved upwards. We were close to the lift that would take us up to my ward and the anaesthetist's destination, and the receptionist had already alighted at her stop. So near yet so far, but my patient needed help right now.

Pulse check, I thought – remembering my training. There was none, though it was confusing as I could definitely feel mine racing. I flattened the head of the trolley, shouting at my patient in an attempt to wake him, willing him to respond. The anaesthetist grabbed an Ambu bag (a bag, mask and valve device used to provide positive-pressure ventilation to patients who are not breathing adequately). He started to 'bag' the man. There was no telephone in sight. I climbed onto the trolley to commence chest compressions when it occurred to me that less than 15 metres away was ICU. I had never set foot in ICU but I knew it was there.

The porter pushed the trolley with me pumping the man's chest. And the anaesthetist helped push the trolley while intermittently providing breaths of oxygen to our lifeless patient, the algorithm of life support banging in my brain.

The doors to ICU opened and I saw a blonde nurse in scrubs calmly beckoning us through the unit to a vacant bed. I watched the slick and efficient way Critical Care staff transferred him onto an ICU bed while simultaneously attaching leads and wires to him. Taking blood, putting drips in, intubating him, connecting fluids.

'Stand back!' He was defibrillated and there it was – the beep, beep, beep of his heart rhythm on the defibrillator monitor. It was mesmerising. I felt as if I was in a dream. I was surrounded by a phenomenal team of skilled medical and nursing staff who seemingly rose up from nowhere and, without question and with such precision, resolved the situation.

In shock, I returned to the ward, several hours after I had left. 'Where have you been?' I explained the detail of my adventure and then had to somehow explain the circumstances to his wife and brother who had arrived to visit.

I took them to ICU where a consultant gently spoke to the shocked family. He relayed information clearly and accurately, having taken in every detail of my account of the events, and he succinctly weaved my story and his personal findings together to update them.

That night I couldn't sleep. I didn't know how my patient was and I was reflecting on the situation and how it could have been avoided. I was working again the next day, so I went in early on Saturday morning – to ICU for an update.

His bed was empty. He must have died. I stood feeling numb, looking at the clean bed space ready and prepared for the next admission.

There was the blonde nurse again, who I now learned was a senior sister. 'Good morning,' she chirped. 'You come to visit Kamal? We moved him into the cubicle, as it was too noisy.' She pointed at the side room and there was my patient, sitting up in bed eating cornflakes. I was astonished. 'Kamal,' she said, 'this is the young nurse who saved your life.'

'Ah, I remember you – thank you very much indeed.' He extended his hand and took mine.

The sister said, 'What happened with you is every nurse's worst nightmare. How are you?' I explained that it was shocking and scary but also extremely exciting, and now I knew that he had made a full recovery I allowed the exhilaration to envelop me.

'What are you doing on Monday?' said the sister. 'We are interviewing for junior staff. You should come for an interview. I think you would fit in well here.'

And that was it. That was the beginning. I passed the interview and never looked back. I never went to ED.

I love it just where I am.

28 November

There is a place, somewhere between life and death. A place created by science and technology. A place made possible by drugs, machinery and know-how. A person is given every chance, metaphorically, to step left or right and head towards their destiny.

This is a place that sometimes makes me feel deeply uncomfortable. Just because we can, doesn't mean we should. Once we have given an injured or ill person every chance and we know for sure they will never recover, the best thing is to stop. Let nature take its course and allow a person to die with comfort and dignity.

Fear, guilt, regret, indecision, love and doubt sometimes mean a family resists allowing a person to die. A person who in some ways has already died. The machinery and medications keep their body alive.

It takes courage to accept, let go and say goodbye. The medical team make a best-interest decision, give the family time to process the information. Then we support the family having time to spend with their loved one, and finally we turn off the machines. This only happens when there is absolutely no chance of meaningful recovery, proven by scans, tests and the assessment and opinion from the entire specialist team. This is never a decision taken lightly.

It is painful to observe the grief and pain. We do all we can to give a patient the best death. I want a family to look back and remember that, despite it being a terrible time, the staff were kind and supportive, and the patient was comfortable and in peace. It is an honour to share these incredible moments with a family.

Covid brings unique challenges. It has its own trajectory and we know it now. When a patient is admitted the team make a plan depending on the individual patient and how ill they are. We know which tests to do and which drugs to give. We learned so much from before and we ensure that we do all we can to support recovery. It is inspiring how medical staff keep up to date on Covid research and hospitals share guidelines on best practice.

One patient was discharged to the ward. She recovered. She was tearful. 'I really thought I was going to die.'

Another patient came off the ventilator and is fine. A few patients have died but mostly they are slowly recovering. This tsunami is less brutal — or perhaps we are more skilled?

Taps are often an issue. Staff yank the lever handles to turn them on or off in a hurry, so the taps often drip — filters are added to reduce infection. There are rules about not putting anything down a sink unless it is water from hand washing. All to reduce infection. The sluice is where we pour any unwanted fluids or water. It is bizarre that both the hot and cold taps provide only lukewarm water. The sink in the store room that is hardly used thunders out hot or cold water.

In some ways nurses are slaves to this pandemic and we are exhausted. The enormous strain on the health service and its staff have been under has largely been forgotten now. People are fed up with Covid and want to get back to normal life. Nurses still pay an annual registration fee of £120 to the NMC (Nursing and Midwifery Council) for the pleasure of being a nurse. Just to be able to work and help people. In light of the extra work and stress it would be lovely to have this annual fee waived — just for this year.

I took a patient to the ward. He had recovered well. Another patient was shouting at a young nurse: 'Get me some water, you stupid girl.'

I intervened: 'Come on. That's not nice. She's not stupid. If you want water, ask nicely.' I was firm but clear and he adjusted his request for water and apologised. The nurse seemed relieved that I had stepped in but, sadly, I am sure that once I left the ward he would continue to speak to her in such a way.

If you ask us how we are, we mostly say we are OK. We are nurses, not victims. I just dream of lying on a beach somewhere incredible.

We are fitted for washable heavy masks that have a filter and tight rubber straps – if we run out of FFP3 masks we need protection. Each nurse will be given their own fitted mask. They are uncomfortable and make your face sore. It's difficult to talk or be heard in them, and we look like we've just stepped out from the *Return of the Jedi* movie set. It is so hard to work while wearing the PPE. I am not a sweaty person but last weekend, after doffing following my shift, my cotton scrub top was wet with perspiration.

Critically ill patients become oedematous (swollen). This can be caused by sodium retention, circulatory impairment, hypotension (low blood pressure) and as a result of fluids given and sepsis. Limbs can become so swollen that rings need to be removed from fingers and arms and legs elevated on pillows. It's a temporary issue during critical illness.

The trust within our team is phenomenal. We work together for hours at a time, day and night. No tension, united in our goal to do the best for our patients. We work, we chat, we laugh and sometimes we cry. One patient said the nurses sweep in like torpedoes, buzzing around and giving meticulous care, never wavering. We might all look the same when in PPE, but those patients who are awake know us well from our eyes.

DECEMBER 2020

5 December

People say, 'It's much better this time.'

Better than what? Better than 15 people dying in one day? Better than working in PPE in the summer with no air con? Better than crying because you are exhausted and frustrated and overwhelmed? It's not better – it's different. Doing something dreadful once is unbearable. But doing it again is also unbearable.

We have seen things that cannot be unseen, yet we keep going. There are nurses who will never quite be the same again. People are still dying and that is never OK. Human life is so precious. Covid has affected everything and everyone, and we wait for the axis to rebalance and normal life to resume.

The other day two people died within 40 minutes of each other. Two people who had a life and family and were struck by Covid. There is also a patient I know. I didn't realise at first, as I didn't recognise him face-down and ventilated. It suddenly hit me when I had to write down his name. This terrible virus has given me fresh perspective on love and life.

Critical Care madness reigns. We are busy but boxes of the most exquisite doughnuts arrive, and staff are there with jam and orange cream on their face, speed-eating their squidgy yumminess.

Fuelled to continue, we continue. Nurses are divided up and distributed like playing cards to the Critical Care units, whether permanent or makeshift, to care for patients with Covid or to care for the usual stream of ill or injured patients. As the hospital aims to continue with elective and emergency surgery, we are stretched way beyond our capacity.

One of my patients looks so much better: freshly shaven, wearing his glasses and tucking into his wife's homemade soup, which was dropped off by a family member. It's good to see a patient looking so well after seeing him so sick.

I helped two nurses clean a patient. One of the support nurses had kindly cleaned all the visors, but she'd used the wrong cleaning wipes, so they were all smeared and we couldn't see a thing. We moved and changed the patient through fogged-up visors, laughing and joking at this ridiculous situation.

Many years ago I cared for a young woman who took off her seatbelt while in a car on the motorway in order to reach into the cool bag on the back seat. Her friend was driving. They were off for a day out together on a hot July day, leaving small children with their fathers.

Her hand grasped the cold bottle of water and, at that very moment, a lorry struck their car sideways. The car was tossed like a ball into the bushes at the edge of the motorway, bouncing against the barrier. The driver was killed instantly, but my patient was retrieved and resuscitated by paramedics before being admitted into Critical Care, where she remained for weeks.

I got to know her family well and, when she left to go for intense rehabilitation for her brain injury, I wondered how she would recover. It was incredible to receive a card last month, eight years later. She had made a complete recovery and hoped I was OK and coping with the pandemic. 'And my mum sends her love,' her card added. She included a photo of her with her family and new baby.

This is a strange stage. Neither the disease mechanism nor treatments for Covid-19 are fully understood. A vaccine is around the corner. Yes, you should have the vaccine. It's a gesture of civil responsibility and anyone who does not have the vaccine should not travel abroad and should pay for their medical bill if they are admitted to hospital with Covid-19. In my opinion, that is. This is not the time to be an 'anti-vaxxer'.

Many Covid patients are diabetic. If they are not diabetic, their blood-glucose levels may become elevated due to critical illness and the large doses of steroids and other drugs they receive. This is called hyperglycaemia. Tight glucose control using insulin is important, as uncontrolled levels can cause secondary issues which can contribute to organ damage and increase the chance of death.

When the body becomes inflamed it triggers an abnormal immune response, which doesn't just attack the virus; it can also affect the body's healthy cells. We try to deal with this appropriately and normalise the blood-glucose level.

There is awesomeness weaving its magic where I work. Nurses are disrupted but doing their absolute best at all times. Nurses from all around the world who speak many different languages. All different but all nurses, and I am honoured and proud to know them. I know them well – sometimes just by looking at their eyes. We should take a moment to realise what we have achieved.

Happy December, everyone.

13 December

Proning is the process of turning someone onto their front to maximise oxygenation. This method is used in Critical Care for patients with acute respiratory distress. Proning is performed on sedated patients and requires a minimum of five trained staff, with an anaesthetist securing the patient's airway and Critical Care nurses managing the turn. It is a perfectly timed and coordinated manoeuvre, and always generates a tangle of drips and wires, and we end up with a crooked bottom sheet. Critical Care nurses can't tolerate a wonky bed sheet.

We have to disconnect and reconnect lines and rejig machinery and equipment. It can be tricky and must be managed well, as a patient can become destabilised, but it does usually improve oxygenation. The patient remains in this position for 12–16 hours and then is turned onto their back again.

A patient's eyes and mouth can become swollen, and we support their face on a doughnut-shaped gel ring. The tubing for ventilation is carefully arranged to reduce pressure. Patients look awful in this position and it's a challenge to nurse them, but it does seem to help Covid patients.

Visitors are not allowed on Covid Critical Care unless a patient is dying, and then only briefly to say goodbye. Pre-Covid, we had adapted to all-day visiting on Critical Care, which was tough on staff who were trying to work while answering endless but understandable questions and comforting shocked and distraught families.

Without visitors it is hard to individualise our patients, to learn about the person they are. A team of staff provide daily family updates and we use FaceTime as a way of connecting patients with their family. Even if a loved one is sedated, at least family can see them. If I talk to a family, I always ask about my patient in order to learn about the person they really are.

On yesterday's night shift we were so short-staffed. Not enough trained staff. Support nurses redeployed from non-ICU areas to help are mostly willing but are unaware of what they don't know. Understandably they are not familiar with intensive-care jargon, the machinery and equipment. It's frustrating for us and overwhelming for them. I am uncomfortable that we have unskilled staff caring for critically ill patients supported by a trained ICU nurse. But we have no choice: we are lucky that these nurses help; otherwise there would be no one. We upskill them as best we can and they learn fast.

I have the best laughs at work – laughing that makes you ache and your eyes water. The kind of laugh that makes you smile and chuckle hours later when you remember it. Mostly, nurses are entirely inappropriate, so some situations cannot be repeated. Those for who English is not their first language have the most wonderful way with pronunciation, and I tease them – only ever out of affection and respect.

Yesterday morning I asked an elderly lady recovering from Covid if she would like a cup of tea. She replied, 'No, darling, thank you. The lovely astronaut brought me one earlier so I am fine.' This made me giggle all day. She is muddled: we look like astronauts, and so she thinks that's who we really are.

There is a man who had an ingrown toenail, which he ignored until the pain was so excruciating that he saw his GP, who prescribed painkillers and antibiotics. He didn't take his entire antibiotic course because after two days his toe felt much better. The infection continued to grow and he was admitted to ICU with sepsis. This week he had his leg amputated just below the knee due to gangrene. It's always important to finish a course of antibiotics.

The nurses from overseas are creating their own Christmas families. Brought together through nationality, trauma, love and restrictions on travel, they are planning and plotting to buy red dresses or shirts online to fulfil their planned Christmas dress code. Some are working, so the Christmas celebrations will be a rolling event as nurses leave for their shift or arrive following their shift on Christmas Day.

I have spent more hours at work this year than anywhere. More hours with this incredible bunch of people than with my family. I have become so close to some of them, and there is a powerful and unbreakable bond between us. It is phenomenal to think we have done this once and now we are doing it again – this time without the clap or the discounts. The war spirit is diminishing. We were celebrated as heroes, but we are forgotten now. Inside us, we carry everything we did and everything we saw.

If this vaccine is successfully rolled out it may be the beginning of the end. I hear endless misinformed opinions at work, on social media and from friends about the shoulds and should-nots. Those who are against the vaccination need to explain how the NHS keeps going. We cannot keep caring for an endless stream of Covid patients. We are running out of everything, and soon we will run out of the people you need the most – Critical Care nurses.

One patient I saw was crying as I was about to leave to go home. She had recently been diagnosed with cancer. Her mastectomy surgery was delayed as she now had Covid. She had almost completed her chemotherapy and wore a scarf to cover her bald head. She wanted to be home; it was her son's birthday. She was recovering but still required oxygen, although she was now Covid-negative. It seems so unfair, cancer and Covid, and one year ago she was fine – a regular working mum and wife. Now her contact with her family is by video call. She told me she has to be upbeat and chatty with them so they won't worry. After the call she just cried.

I went Christmas shopping this week. The streets and shops did not have the usual hustle and bustle, even if the Christmas lights and music were abundant. Maybe I just noticed more this year.

21 December

It's 4 a.m. I can't sleep and this email is late. I worked 14 hours yesterday and I am so tired, but still I cannot sleep.

I have a rich insight into how it really is. It matters a lot that we seem to be permanently short of drugs, equipment and various supplies. Some hospitals have run out of oxygen. In my wildest dreams I did not know a hospital could run out of oxygen – it never occurred to me.

Not enough staff and a lack of appropriately trained staff. We were on the edge before the pandemic. Does it matter? To me and all the incredible nurses and healthcare professionals, it matters so much, as we have to keep on, accept the situation and do our absolute best – every second of the day and night.

I don't think the general public really have any idea what Critical Care nurses do and what we see. We feel guilty if we don't work, exhausted if we do. We are under enormous strain but continue to march forward, but at least the end is – possibly – in sight.

Sometimes it's impossible to process. To work in such a way, return home, walk through your own front door and switch back. To come back down to earth from the planet that has just owned and consumed you for hours. To morph suddenly back into the other person again.

We are so short-staffed that we work on our days off. There is nowhere to go and not much to do, so nurses may as well earn a bit extra. Christmas hampers and treats are arriving, and the war-torn nurses are thrilled to see the treasures wrapped within ribbon and cellophane. Now that we are in Tier 4, with Christmas apparently cancelled, these gifts mean even more.

The best moment this week was when I asked a consultant to help clean a patient who had profuse diarrhoea in the extreme. The patient was sedated and unaware that two nurses and a very senior anaesthetist were washing him, cleaning the bed and mopping the floor. This took almost an hour. The consultant was gagging despite the FFP3 mask and visor, but we jokingly said that we assessed her as competent to clean up poo and laughed at her poor constitution. Nurses have to be resistant to the various smells we are exposed to. We all have a scent we like the least – for me it's the smell of burnt flesh.

'How do you do this?' was the comment I heard from beneath the mask. I reminded the consultant to be mindful about prescribing laxatives in future. 'Never again,' came the reply.

We lost brothers this week, within 40 minutes of each other. They died in different areas of Covid ICU – so sad for their sister going back and forth between them during her pre-booked, allocated time slots to be with her siblings for the last time.

It's busy, so busy. Tempers are frayed and fuses are short. We wait for the world to come back. My colleagues are bruised. Teamwork remains excellent mostly, but there has been some friction, only because we are totally and utterly exhausted. This is a strange stage. A vaccine is around the corner. We have learned so much yet so very little too.

I am challenged on many levels. Exceptional leadership and resilience are required to do this job on Critical Care – even more so on a Covid Critical Care. Ensuring professional and safety standards are met, supporting staff, caring for patients and coordinating admissions, transfers and discharges. Providing expertise, help, advice and connecting with the myriad of people who 'keep the show on the road'. Negotiating and standing up for patients and staff, and running around to find the plastic connection that attaches thing one to thing two, as the suppliers have changed but no one remembered to check if the product is compatible with connecting equipment! It's tough and tiring and stressful.

We have many patients suffering from alcoholic liver disease (ALD). The liver starts to fail after years of excessive drinking and the result can be fatal. This infliction seems to be more common and patients are becoming younger. I nursed a woman years ago, a frequent patient: patched up, discharged and re-admitted a few months later. She was always bright yellow from jaundice, her abdomen swollen from an accumulation of fluid (ascites) that needed to be drained or the build-up would rise, squashing her lungs and making her breathless.

I was in the park with my own child a few years later when a young woman pushing a toddler on a swing reminded me who she was. She had finally recovered and was now a wife and mother. This woman beat alcoholism, but Covid is affecting many people with alcohol dependency, their damaged bodies too frail to resist its vicious grip.

Merry Christmas to you all, and thank you for your endless support. We will be working throughout Christmas and the New Year, every second of the day and night, to do our best for our patients. Please remember us and that, despite inadequate funding and staffing, we laugh, have fun and somehow perform miracles.

23 December

'Please bring me a bottle of water. It's hell and I think I may die soon ... I also need a hug too, please. If they haven't run out.' This is a text message I received at 5 a.m. from one of my nurses. She got water, a hug and a chocolate croissant.

We keep going.

As a child, I would run down the up escalator for fun. I often think of that now, as it's how this feels. I need to get off and press the large red emergency stop button. But it doesn't seem to work, so we keep running.

And so it continues, with no end in sight. We escalate into other areas.

The cotton PPE gowns became paper gowns, and now they are plastic. Our scrubs are soaked in sweat, and I feel the perspiration run down my body beneath the plastic. It's like wearing a wetsuit, a layer of water keeping you warm. The white shrouds we use for the dead bodies are made of the same material as the blue gowns. We are working in shrouds.

The death is disturbing. People have a right to die if they have reached that point. Today I had to fight for a patient's right to die. Her pre-existing health challenges were an issue, but add Covid to the mix and quality survival was extremely unlikely and, after 52 days, it was time to allow her to be left in peace. It was deemed that she would not recover from her multi-organ failure (heart, lung, renal and hepatic failure). She was unconscious and had been for days. It was time. It was tough to tell her daughter on the phone that her mum had just died. No easy way to break this news.

Clotting and bleeding are an issue in Covid patients. Pulmonary embolism (PE) and deep vein thrombosis (DVT) are diagnosed when a blood clot lodges itself in the lung or leg. We measure a patient's blood results and clinical signs carefully for clues as to whether this has or is likely to occur, and we prescribe appropriate treatment. Some blood results correlate with disease severity and we act accordingly.

Working in this way is hard. Every pod has a large trolley with drawers containing an orderly supply of the most-used equipment and drugs: tubes, syringes, gauze, needles, fluids, connectors, drip lines, filters. The list is endless, but each individual pod has its own storage area in a different place and in a different order. No one has the time to create a system. The current system is how it is in the individual pods 1, 2, 3 or 4.

The runner who stocks the trolley has no idea what most of the items are used for, so it is not surprising that I find the mouth swabs in the same pot as the insulin syringes. I turn in circles daily, as I can't find what I need or the drawer is empty, so I shout, leaning out through the door like a baby demanding to be fed, 'Can someone get me an HME!' A helpful person will go to find the missing item – in this case a Heat and Moisture Exchanger – but, as they often have no idea what it is they are looking for, it takes them ages and they return with something entirely different. I heard that one helper had to google the item. Like last time, by the time we stop the helpers will have learned what everything is for and where to find it.

Perhaps if we had all been quicker, stricter and sooner with the mask wearing and social distancing we might have beaten this, cut it off in its tracks. Or maybe not. But we will all leave 2020 with bruising from what this year has done to everyone, and even though the damage to nurses is immeasurable, it is what we do and our purpose. For others who were slaughtered, it will leave psychological, emotional, financial, social, educational and literal scars.

Amidst the madness and mayhem there are those unforgettable moments. A patient who grabs your arm, squeezes it and says thank you, or holds your hand tight as they are scared and we are their anchor and safety for that moment. Being told you make a difference. And there are the hilarious comments. A patient asked me, 'Am I on the right road for Tunbridge Wells?'

I nursed an opera singer once. He was elderly, frail, breathless and in need of respiratory support. I explained how the CPAP (continuous positive airway pressure) machine with its tight mask worked. How it expanded his lungs to help him breathe, thus improving his blood oxygenation. 'Like singing,' he said. He asked me to help him out of bed. I held his catheters and drips and arranged the monitor leads while he wobbled, stood up and, holding onto the bed rail and my arm, he sang an Ella Fitzgerald song – belting it out at full volume. Suddenly, a group of medics gathered around the bed to listen. The oxygen saturation recordings on the monitor settled within normal limits.

When he'd finished singing and bowed to the applause, I settled him back into bed. A young man appeared, shook his hand and said, 'That was incredible. I have been sitting with my grandmother who is dying. She used to love that song. Thank you.'

These moments are the ones that embed in me; my reasons for doing this in the first place.

We just have to ride the storm.

Boxing Day, 2020

It's been a bizarre year and none of us anticipated the curve ball that launched itself at us. But look at what we've achieved.

In the midst of tragedy we're often finding a way to get people through this year, and there are people raising a glass with loved ones this Christmas who wouldn't be here if it wasn't for our dedication, expertise, compassion and sheer resilience.

Patients are moved around. From A&E to the ward, to another ward, to theatre, to Critical Care. And the dentures, glasses and phone go missing – they will turn up, though maybe not this week. Those favourite blue slippers *shall* turn up at some point. Usually we are more organised, but we are focused on the business of the patient. Property is the last thing on our mind.

Many times I have rummaged through a patient's belong-ings, searching for a particular item. Property mostly includes socks, trainers, phone charger, jacket, bus pass, keys, towel, hairbrush and always scrunched-up tissues. But there are sometimes other items. Packets of white powder, half-eaten chocolate bars, suspenders, crotchless knickers, hordes of cash – possibly tucked into the lining of a jacket. One man was admitted with 11 iPhones in his bag, and another with duct tape and rope.

We never know what buried treasure we will find. Paramedics scoop up a person's property at the scene of an accident, and once, when I was going through a bag looking for door keys for a patient's wife, I pulled out a blood-soaked T shirt and jeans that had been cut off by the ambulance crew. I found the keys, a smashed iPad and ... an index finger. My patient wasn't missing a finger.

We admitted a patient from an oxygen-deprived hospital. The transfer from A to B was meticulous, well planned and organised, but still the process destabilised this young woman who had recently completed a course of chemotherapy. With her immune system blown to pieces, she succumbed to Covid. It took an hour to synchronise her ventilator settings and steady her heart rate with drugs then defibrillation. Then she was stable and the monitor and ventilator displayed more favourable measurements and patterns.

The pandemic slaves continue to work hard. Dealing with the daily carnage. Stretched thin to create more Covid space. We wrap ourselves in knots while manoeuvring around the limited space between the beds. Cables, wires, tubes, lines. We duck under, climb over, bashing our PPE-clad heads on pumps or machines. We laugh as the ventilator support clamp hooks up with our visor and we are suspended for a second while another nurse unthreads us.

So few nurses means we have less time to be as thorough as we would like; we do as much as we can with negative time. We document what we need to and the clock has turned back to task allocation. One nurse does all the drugs, another records the observations. We take on a role within our pod, our team. This is team-building in the extreme. We are each other's silent support.

Before, we would just care for our one patient and help our colleagues when required. Task allocation makes working slicker but experience tells us this spreads infection, so it is not the way we usually work, pre-Covid. We share patients now because there is no choice. Far from ideal for anyone.

It's Christmas but our patients have no visitors. We play Christmas music loudly and do the PPE dance when time allows. It's so weird and not how we usually celebrate with our patients. Christmas is forgotten, as it's too busy and the surreal environment does not feel Christmassy at all.

A man died but he had no name band on. Hospital policy is that every patient has two name bands detailing their name, date of birth and MRN (medical records number). A red band alerts us to an individual's allergy. At least I recognised this man's face. I had nursed him many times and had spoken to his daughter on the phone. We have to cut corners and it is not OK, but there is zero choice. An excellent and experienced Critical Care nurse will progress their patient, work with the physio, pharmacist, medical team — the entire MDT (multi-disciplinary team) plan and execute high-standard, progressive care. We have specialists in everything. All with their individual expertise. We always give our best.

Now the approach is different; it has to be. We tread water, we are at war, we prioritise our care, and despite staffing levels we somehow open another area and the staff-to-patient ratio is further reduced.

As I've mentioned before, our nurses come from all over the world. We had a Spanish patient who didn't speak English, but we had a Spanish nurse. We literally meet our patients' every need. A Chinese lab assistant kindly came to our unit to translate the Mandarin of a Chinese patient whose English was limited.

Brexit and Covid will surely decimate our Critical Care nurse population. It takes several years acquiring qualifications and experience to be competent and skilled enough to safely care for any unstable, critically ill individual. These nurses can't be plucked out of thin air to operate a ventilator. As I have said before, this is a skill that most doctors don't have. The NHS is so lucky and honoured to have such a plethora of highly skilled, brilliant warrior nurses who are dealing with the Covid bomb.

The plan changes as the situation develops. It's tough and is predicted to get tougher. Christmas gift bags, treats and hampers arrive. Do not underestimate how much these mean to us.

This note was left for me to pass on:

I arrived at work for the night shift on Christmas Eve, feeling sad, thinking of my husband alone at home, feeling anxious about the carnage that awaited me, feeling apprehensive about our staffing, feeling the constant worry that the current situation is not going away any time soon and in all likelihood is going to get worse. I see a few colleagues sitting in the staff room, their faces reflecting the exhaustion they feel after another 12.5-hour shift with not enough nurses. The usual Christmas cheer muted by fatigue and the knowledge that, like everyone else, we won't be seeing loved ones on our days off this year.

There is a gift bag for me. Glancing inside I see a bunch of goodies and know that wonderful, amazing people are still on the case of supporting nurses. Helping, supporting and caring for us. My eyes fill with tears and I go and sit in the loo, take a moment to have a quick cry. I cry for myself. Tired, frightened, worried and still processing everything that we dealt with in the first surge. I cry for my colleagues who have been fighting this war for what feels like for ever and who share all my own fears and anxieties. I cry for all the people we couldn't save, the ones who died and the ones who will die. I cry for the non-Covid patients who won't get the treatment or care they otherwise would. I cry for the people who have lost loved ones and jobs and businesses and those who won't see family this Christmas.

But I also cry tears of gratitude. For the people who, despite their own challenges, still think of, help and support the nurses. These people are amazing and I thank them from the bottom of my heart. We carry on because this is our job, this is what nurses do. We couldn't walk away even if we wanted to. You could walk away in a heartbeat but you don't and that's incredible.

Please know how much we appreciate everything you do and have done for us.

Thank you.

JANUARY 2021

2 January

Critical Care nurses are a precious and valuable resource. This Covid explosion cannot be beaten without us. We are on our knees. I honestly don't know how we keep going. It's like hell. I could never have imagined it would be like this, and it keeps getting worse. A war zone, fire-fighting, and the invisible beast is around every corner. All NHS staff are standing up and facing this full on. From porters to consultants, we stand tall and strong.

Ambulance after ambulance arrives with patients fighting for breath. With a history of a persistent cough and lethargy, they are hypoxic, have a temperature and a raised D-dimer (a blood test to identify blood clots) – we know what the swab result will say. The hospital desperately tries to shuffle beds around to accommodate them. There are queues outside the Emergency Department. Sick patients come from their homes as well as those transferred from other areas or hospitals. All in desperate need to share the dwindling beds and resources. I would joke that we need bunk beds.

A heroic effort is once again underway to enact surge plans. Management have cancelled operations to free up staff and equipment. It is unmanageable, unsustainable and truly scary.

More wards become temporary ICUs. Yet as quickly as we free up more beds, they are filled – but we do not have the staff to care for the patients. We do our best, prioritise while thinking on our feet. We work together as a team.

We use portable ventilators and anaesthetic machines, the kind of ventilators used for operations and transfers, not intended for the long-term ventilation of sick patients. We have to learn in an instant how to operate them. My eyes search for the button or knob I need, each different brand of ventilator having them in a different place.

It's not just Covid patients. Heart attacks, falls from ladders and down the stairs, car accidents, bike accidents, explosions, self-harm. Patients with cancer who need urgent treatment. Those who drink or take recreational drugs in excess; they too fill our beds. And those who don't have Covid but are suffering from the consequences of Covid need our help and care, too.

A patient who, while walking his dog, had a cardiac arrest, was resuscitated by a passer-by and then a paramedic. He woke up in hospital, confused and disoriented, but alive and apparently without any long-lasting damage. He was petrified and desperately trying to get out of bed to escape. He had no reliable cognitive function and was pulling out lines and tubes. It took five nurses to hold him while he punched and fought us off, and then we chemically restrained him to keep him safe and manage his recovery.

Much of my time is spent reassuring his terrified wife and teenage daughter on the phone. We are running on limited staff and this man required an hour's attention from five nurses. There were four nurses left to observe the other fourteen critically ill patients, and only one of those nurses was Critical Care trained, and she is pregnant.

Covid now is a different beast. The tsunami that hit us before, hits again but from a different direction, a different angle. It's like being pelted with stones with no time to duck.

The NHS is incredible, my team are phenomenal and – somehow – we keep going. A nurse came to help from another hospital and commented on the superb teamwork.

The number of Covid patients changes each hour with admissions, transfers and deaths. We are way beyond our regular capacity. It's hard to look into our patients' eyes, to see their fear. We try to be tender and reassure them. Those on respiratory support, who cannot talk, look at our faces, their eyes burning through, trying to communicate. We mind-read and answer their questions as best we can. They want to know if they will survive, and many do because they receive the absolute best care, despite everything.

Not since the Second World War have we seen death and suffering on such a level without a sign of it ending. Critical Care staff are the soldiers and fighter pilots, and we are also suffering. We arrive early, leave late, forgo breaks and often carry around a full bladder. Always thirsty, frequently hungry, tired, overwhelmed and mesmerised by this ongoing attack.

Many of our staff now have Covid or are self-isolating. The rest of us are exhausted but still come to work. We all feel enormous pressure to be at work, because if we are not there, that is one less nurse. On days off we feel guilty and displaced and want to be at work. When we're at work we want to be at home.

Weird and wonderful happens on Critical Care. My heart has been full of love and of pain. I have laughed until I ache and cried for hours. Being a nurse devours but enriches me. I have seen life, death, tragedy, love, horror, kindness, compassion, hope and bravery.

However, in this world of unpredictability, we are privileged, as we have seen incredible, phenomenal and beautiful – unseen by anyone else.

9 January

Lockdown, Tier 3, Tier 4, Tier 5 … and still we keep going.

Some hospitals have seriously low levels of piped oxygen. The ambient oxygen in the air from all we are using is at a dangerous measurement; it is a fire hazard. Sometimes I wonder if the staff are at risk from breathing in air enriched with oxygen. Maybe in the future, healthcare workers will be suffering from some respiratory condition blamed on the effects of this, like asbestosis.

We are running out of everything – we are running out of resilience. We have to be careful when using some electrical equipment, as it overloads the power supply in an area not designed to function as Critical Care, where we have scores of power points, oxygen and air ports.

Now, when switching a patient between two different ventilation methods, which can be many times a day (unless you can find an adapter or have an oxygen cylinder to hand), you quickly unplug the white hose and switch over to the other piece of equipment, shoving the second hose back into the port until you hear the familiar hiss. All done in a cramped space, leaning and stretching. The bruises that appear from the bumps and knocks get compared in the changing room.

Covid creates a dense white shadow in both lungs on a patient's chest X-ray. Blood tests and clotting results are abnormal. Patients are short of breath, have a high temperature and feel ill. This is the general clinical pattern. There are different presentations too that can be initially confusing. We endlessly aim to give the best care we can, but it is becoming increasingly difficult, as we are so stretched and diluted.

We spoke with a man today who has just been diagnosed with leukaemia. We discussed his prognosis and a plan of care based on his CT scan, chest X-ray and blood results, which confirm he is Covid-positive. The reality is: if he is ventilated, he will probably die; if he is not, he will probably die. 'What can I do to help myself?' he asked.

There are no words to explain the madness. I have not stopped for 14 hours. I cannot talk or think or even walk properly once I finish my shift. I tried to reassure a nurse caring for three patients on ventilators. 'I don't know about ventilators,' she said. We now offer sub-optimal care, only due to a lack of knowledge and experience, not a lack of caring or willingness. Senior staff try their best to guide and teach our fabulous support crew, and it breaks my heart. It is hard to leave and go home. When I leave my colleagues and patients I feel I am betraying them. There are not enough Critical Care nurses.

It's raw and real and I genuinely don't know how nurses will come back from this. I am strong and it is breaking me.

We still laugh. We are still inappropriate. We joke and tease and care for each other. We cry, together or alone. I hug nurses I have never met before but who have helped us and with whom we stand shoulder to shoulder. At the end of the shift we are united in survival and yet we delay going home. Crossing the threshold from hospital to home is so hard. There is this magnetic force field that implores you to stay just a little bit longer. Unlike the troops in a battle, we get to go home after a day or night at war on the front line. I am not sure if this is helpful or not.

The monumental physical and emotional load is hard to bear, and it is getting harder. The pandemic slaves continue on. I spent five minutes I didn't have chatting with a single mum. She was worried about her young son who was being cared for by a neighbour, as her family all live in Scotland. Too busy to chat with a patient is a place I never thought I would get to. During our conversation I saw that her ECG monitoring cables were on back to front, her arterial line had not been calibrated, her catheter bag was overflowing, and her IV hydrocortisone drip line was two days out of date.

Sub-standard care delivered by inexperienced non-ICU staff. It's not their fault.

Please do nothing that may require you to come into hospital. Sometimes it cannot be avoided, but after half a bottle of wine, climbing a ladder is never a great idea. That tree branch can wait ... Don't drive your car fast, don't ride a motorbike, wear a helmet, don't spray toxic waterproof solution on your boots in an enclosed space, don't leave a pan of oil on the stove and forget it's there, and please don't take recreational drugs that may well be made with ingredients your heart cannot cope with. Don't admonish a fellow driver who cuts you up – that driver may have a knife. And if you are unsteady on your feet, please don't go out in the pouring rain.

The NHS say that, throughout the pandemic, the NHS is open for business for those who need it, so anyone requiring care can receive it. But hospitals are running on empty. In the current climate, when there are not enough beds or staff and the queues for ED are long, we may not be able to offer you the care you deserve.

Critical Care has no beds left, but somehow magic happens and the senior clinical team, bed manager, site team and Critical Care matrons juggle and manoeuvre, and somehow find a bed.

16 January

It's worse than it was in March when it first began. It's tough and, true to form, people all get sick at the same time. One day patients are sick and unstable, and the next an entire group of patients are clutching onto life and threatening to die simultaneously. A&E are delivering yet more patients, or the outreach team are packaging up a deteriorating patient from the ward and transporting them, freshly intubated, to whichever makeshift Critical Care area has space.

There is a craziness in swapping beds around in such a cramped space – it's like a game of Twister, transferring a patient from a ward bed to an ICU bed. Sometimes we don't bother if the patient is sick or unstable, so all our beds and specialised mattresses are in the wrong place. Two patients are jammed into a room intended for one patient and, once you add in the equipment, it becomes impossible. Nurses need to be flexible and agile to negotiate the obstacles around the beds.

Winter is usually busy with seasonal flu, slips and trips, mental-health issues. It's always worse in the winter and, if the weather is bad and there is ice on the road, admissions increase exponentially.

I don't sleep well, as the merry-go-round of the day contin-ues in my brain; it penetrates my dreams. For now, there is no escape.

I cared for a young woman who recovered from Covid but has heart damage as a result. She already suffered from hypertension, but the effects of Covid have caused irreversible damage to her heart – she needed a bed on our Coronary Care Unit (CCU) but none was available. One minute a high-powered lawyer, now a vulnerable patient whose life expectancy has suddenly diminished.

The ever-worsening pandemonium, and we are exhausted. We are spoilt with hot meals and sweet treats donated by the local community, who lovingly bake and drop off trays of delicious, mouth-watering produce. But we are broken and shocked and dismayed that even now, after all we have done, there is no mention of a pay rise, bonus or anything.

I write down the names of the staff on my shift, as I have no idea who some of them are. I know my own crew and I am struck by the awesomeness of our team, some of the most flexible and resourceful people I have ever known. We are hanging on by our fingertips, so we bond fast, and each shift a temporary family is created – different nurses from different areas, and I get to know their beautiful eyes that communicate so much. At the end of the day, when people change out of their sweat-soaked scrubs and you see their face and hair and smile, you get a glimpse of who they really are.

The legacy of this pandemic will destroy 2021 and continue to destroy the NHS and its staff. For years we have been on the edge, working within an underfunded, badly managed, abused system. We are shipwrecked and there are no rescue boats coming our way; that's how it feels. If this pandemic keeps going we will get to a point where if you turn up sick at hospital there may be no nurse, no doctor to see you, and no bed if you need one now or in any meaning-ful timeframe.

23 January

There is an emergency body storage facility – so many deaths together are difficult for the mortuary to manage. It is full.

When a person dies the family are usually with the patient, or a nurse will stay with them. I would never let someone die alone. In Covid times visiting is strictly limited but, as much as we can, we try to allow two members of the family to be with their loved one at the end of their life. This must be dreadful: in full PPE and with a time limit – impossible to imagine. If you love someone, you need to be with them. Most families understand, but it doesn't stop it being total agony for them. Some have seen death via a video link. I cannot even imagine how this is, especially as people are not used to a Critical Care environment, with tubes, drips, wires, monitors and a cacoph-ony of bleeping and shrill alarms.

Ventilation is an intervention of last resort. We don't intu-bate a patient unless we need to protect their airway or support their breathing to improve oxygenation. There is some support for the idea that early ventilation is helpful in Covid, before a patient tires. We explain the procedure if we can, and I will hold their hand as anaesthetic drugs send them 'to sleep'. When you hold a patient's hand, they always squeeze you tightly.

With Covid, the entire body is affected: heart, lungs, kidneys, brain, liver, blood vessels. We investigate, prognosticate, examine and make a plan, which is reviewed and updated, every second if required.

Having fewer staff means it cannot be seconds or even minutes. We are spread thinly and we adjust, change and alter when we can – not soon enough, and because there are not enough appropriately trained nurses it's impossible to give the very best care, and that's the hardest thing of all. ICU nurses are meticulous but our attention to detail cannot be the same now.

We need to be alert. Nurses learn on the job. We have staff helping who work in primary schools or are dental nurses. We have nurses from clinics or endoscopy, areas that have zero connection with events and procedures that occur in a Critical Care environment. Last night I asked a young woman in scrubs to prepare a drug infusion for me. She happily went to find everything and was back moments later with the requested items. I asked if she would mix and prepare the drugs, but she couldn't. 'I'm actually a hairdresser,' she said. She did help – she was willing and amazing – but this is not appropriate on any level, though it is how we have to roll right now.

During the second wave, the army came to help, which made a massive difference – willing to help, they brought fresh enthusiasm and a sense of humour. A young man helped me wash a body and only told me after the event that this was the first dead person he had ever seen. Another told me of the horrors he had witnessed in Afghanistan – it depended where they had been deployed to.

Senior staff keep up to date with the latest advice and research, doing what they know to be best for the Covid patient. ICU nurses alert medical staff about improvements and deterioration. Different teams are emerging to prone or transfer ventilated patients to MRI, CT or another establishment.

Some of the nurses are petrified. One junior nurse was crying at the beginning of the day. 'I can't do this,' she said. When I see our environment with fresh eyes, I understand her fear. I am familiar with and understand this place, and it still scares me.

There is nothing I've experienced that compares with this. It's astonishing that it's OK for NHS staff to just keep going and going and going. Thankfully, the majority of people support us and are grateful for what we do and the difference we make.

I am helping a nurse turn the head of a proned patient. They adopt the front crawl position and every four hours we turn their head to the other side and adjust the position of their arms, one up, one down. I look at the nurse's masked face. She is so gentle with the unconscious man, ensuring his face is as comfortable as possible in this impossible position.

Eyes with immaculate precision eyeliner glance back at me. Her dark brown eyes, truly beautiful and refreshing amid the chaos we are submerged in. She smiles at me, herself broken but still smiling, the powerful urge to see her family in Greece suppressed at work to focus and care.

Proning may help oxygenation but many of these patients suffer from pressure sores to their face. Their eyes and lips swell, their forehead and chin may develop blisters – delicate skin that is face down, with an endotracheal tube and naso-gastric tube secured in their mouth or nose. Snot, saliva and tears covering their face due to gravity's pull – we wipe or suction the fluid away when we can. Hair becomes matted with sweat, blood, spit and vomit. We comb hair back. When the world was normal, we would wash our patients' hair.

Some patients have significant complications. Some cata-strophically collapse and we pull them back from the brink over and over again. Some will fight on and recover; many will not.

The day is threaded through with the regular, everyday occurrences we're all used to. The phone rings non-stop, the printer runs out of ink, a family call to complain. The fire alarm is tested, the floors are cleaned, the pharmacy porter delivers the medication, transport is ordered to transfer a patient to another hospital. The day to day still happens but, hidden away in borrowed spaces, Critical Care works its magic.

Critical Care nursing is about anatomy, physiology, compassion, being practical and adaptable, with flexible communication skills, grit and a huge, huge heart – and a passion for cake and biscuits.

28 January

Jonathan Silver has written another brilliant piece about the pandemic and its effects on the hospital:

'So it went up, and up, and now we're at the "bumpy top". We are at a sustained peak of demand, where the infection numbers are apparently going down again, but the pressure on our services remains as yet unchanged. We have not been able to close any temporary Critical Care areas: we still have a Critical Care department with (by my count) 230 per cent its usual capacity, although we don't have the staff to have all those beds open all the time ...

'Soon, the numbers of patients will start coming down, lagging a couple of weeks behind the drop in infections. As the pressure comes off, the most important thing we as a health service need to do is manage that transition so that exhausted staff get a break. We will be expected to get straight back on the accelerator and face the huge backlog of planned treatment. And this is the right thing to do, but if we do not strike a balance and give everyone a breather, we will utterly break a whole generation of clinical staff – and that's those who aren't already broken. In fact, every step about managing the pandemic is about finding balance: usually the balance of risk ...'

For instance, Jonathan says that one of the most vital pieces of ICU equipment is the syringe pump, 'delivering life-supporting drugs at an extremely precise rate; it's not unusual for a critically ill patient to need eight or ten running at the same time. These "smart pumps" are surprisingly sophisticated; you turn it on, enter the name of the drug you want to give, then the weight of the patient, then the prescribed dose. It measures the syringe you've put in, and it calculates exactly how fast to run that syringe to achieve that dose, as well as noticing and stopping you if you accidentally enter an extra zero.

'As we created more ICU beds this winter, our pumps got spread more and more thinly. The government provided us with more pumps, but very basic ones that don't do any calculating at all. We spread the smart pumps out as best we could, so that no bed ended up with too many basic ones, particularly for the most critical drugs. Meanwhile, we took away all the smart pumps that we could get away with taking, to keep as a stock buffer to allow us to open the next emergency area safely. By taking smart pumps away, we were forcing staff to use the basic ones, at a much-increased risk of making a calculation error, while keeping a stash of perfectly good smart pumps in our store not being used. But if we didn't have that stash, we would end up opening the next area with no smart pumps at all. Or there might never be a next area to open, and the risk is for noth- ing.'

He says there is no right answer, 'just a lot of hand-wring- ing and self-examination. The key is not to make these decisions in isolation ...'

30 January

'How is work?' people ask. How can that question possibly be answered?

This isn't my work anymore. It's fire-fighting in a sand storm. I don't know this place. This place of madness where the ratio of patients to nurses doesn't add up, and there are so many helpers it takes a while to learn who is who and who knows what.

It's truly hard, especially when you know that many of the patients will die. Some survive, but once someone is admitted to Critical Care they are already in a precarious position. It's like working aboard the *Titanic*. This ship will sink.

We are exhausted. Brightly coloured scrub hats and home-made cake really help, but our faces are sore and our hands hurt. We are dehydrated from the sweat and tears we shed. We are displaced, dislocated and fatigued. Spring 2020 was the dress rehearsal – how could it be worse than that? But it is, and there is no sign yet of it abating.

Many patients are diabetic. Some manage their condition well; some do not, and are non-compliant with medication and managing their eating pattern. Many patients require an infusion of insulin, which helps control blood glucose. Critically ill patients often require steroids, and these can cause a drug-induced increase in blood glucose, which is transient and reversible. It's important to maintain a patient's blood glucose within normal limits – mortality is associated with untreated hyperglycaemia. It seems that the majority of

Covid patients require insulin, and each shift I am endlessly preparing syringes ready for use.

A bed was empty for a moment. I helped transfer a patient from a trolley onto this clean bed. The mattress was still warm from the dead body we removed ten minutes earlier. Random helpers clean around the pod at speed to ensure it is as clean as possible for the next patient. And if we can't find a mop or a domestic, nurses are on their hands and knees cleaning the floor.

Our patients are vulnerable, and with so few qualified and appropriately trained nurses, we need to move between many different patients. This increases the chance of spreading infection. We try our best to maintain infection-control stand-ards, but with so few staff it is sometimes impossible. A Covid patient or any critically ill patient is sick, and the complication of sepsis makes them sicker.

The limitations we are working under are so challenging. There are different levels of resilience. It is not just the Covid patients. We segregate non-Covid critically ill patients. There is an escalation area. When I went there late one evening to check on a nurse I was concerned about, the lights had been dimmed. At first glance, the area looked like a car park, beds jammed into spaces where there wasn't really space. If there is an oxygen supply, there is room for a bed.

This is a Covid nightmare. How do we keep up? Patients deserve the best care but we are forced to cut corners. There is no choice – there are too few ICU nurses. We are not afraid of hard work. We cannot do our job to the usual high standards but there are good moments. I brushed and plaited a young girl's hair, and everyone who walked by the bed space commented. I spoon-fed a patient strawberry yoghurt – these are the moments of normal. A patient called me over and said that he didn't like this pub because he hadn't been served any beer – I'm with him!

Out of the blue, one long-term, non-Covid patient had a cardiac arrest. He received immediate rescue protocol and resuscitation from our usual team. We performed chest compressions, defibrillation, and administered emergency drugs as per the ALS (Advanced Life Support) algorithm imprinted on our brains. Resuscitation lasted for over an hour.

He died, despite our best efforts, and we all cried. Doctors, nurses and even the receptionist. We stood around the body, amid the detritus these emergency situations bring: trolleys around the bed spilling over with the leftover contents of emergency intubation and cannulation; discarded pillows and empty packaging on the floor, removed hurriedly in order to perform CPR, and empty syringes on the bed.

Blood, sutures, suction tubing, wires, Elastoplast tape rolls, plastic gloves, discarded machinery, half-drawn blue curtains, monitors bleeping and displaying the flatline (asystole, when there's no heart beat), and the regular green Waters circuit (a breathing system used to manually deliver oxygen) lay next to the patient's face. A familiar scene following an emergency.

A dead man we were all fond of and a team of PPE-clad staff crying. A strange sight to see but only witnessed by each other, and we all understood the release of grief, which wasn't only for this one gentleman.

A West Indian patient with fruity language was given one of our cotton scrub hats to contain his wild dreadlocks. He looked fabulous, sitting up in bed cross-legged, wearing a bright yellow hat covered in pineapples. I asked if I could take a photo. 'Na! Fuck off!' So I didn't. The image, however, was a great one, and is firmly lodged in my mind.

It's fast-paced, noisy, excellent, scary, strange, overwhelming and totally unrelenting. We are shattered and, for many of us, it is hard to engage with anything else at all until this is over or we are done.

*   *   *

It is easy to trip over leads, cables and wires around a Critical Care bed space. There are machines and pumps and monitors that take up space. I almost tripped over the long metal chain that shackled together a prisoner, who is a patient, and a prison officer. My patient is sick but awake and is a 'flight risk'.

This patient required complex treatment for a long-standing health issue. On-site healthcare facilities at most prisons are limited, so inmates are admitted to hospital for the care they require. Prison officers remain at their side at all times. Sometimes this seems crazy when the patient is sedated or unconscious with a handcuff on their wrist, but there are strict rules in place.

Sometimes these patients are guarded by police officers who are there to protect the patient, perhaps from further assault or self-harm, or to arrest or talk to a patient once they come to. They add to the clutter at the bedside, but are always friendly and polite, and at times I feel bad when they keep jumping out of the way to give me immediate and direct access to the patient.

I remember nursing a man brought in from prison after he'd been in a fight. He was septic from a huge abscess on his arm. I was cleaning his wound and we'd been chatting away for a while: patient, nurse and two prison officers – an eclectic group of people laughing and chatting together. The patient asked, 'Do you want to know why I'm in prison?' I did want to know, of course, but I would never ask, and on occasions when you hear their crime, you often prefer not to know.

He told me he was arrested for breaking and entering. He broke into people's homes, which was pre-planned, or opportunistic if he saw an open window. Once he had sneaked into a house while the front door was open, he hid until the family were asleep and then relieved them of phones, laptops and cash before letting himself out. This man was funny and friendly. I told him that I enjoyed chatting with him but that 'I wouldn't want to encounter you in my home. If I was burgled, it would devastate me.'

He then told me the security measures I should put in

place to minimise the chance of this happening to me. 'If someone can afford posh front-door furniture,' he said, 'they have decent stuff to nick inside.'

He advised me on the locks, hinge bolts and London bar (steel door reinforcer) to buy. These items still secure my home today. Who could be better to offer advice on home security than a burglar?

He was thrilled when I found the source of his sepsis. It was the tip of a fingernail embedded in his wound, which saved him a trip to theatre for a debridement (a procedure where infected or necrotic tissue is removed from a wound, which is then thoroughly cleaned and dressed).

We often have the police or prison officers on our unit. The general public often complain about the police, but all my experience has been good. Theirs is not an easy job. Sometimes they are spat at, kicked and sworn at by patients. I remember when a man was admitted after suffering from a traumatic amputation after being hit by a car. A policeman chased him down the road as he was running away from the scene with blood pouring from his shoulder. The young policeman wrapped the inebriated patient's shoulder in his jacket to stem the blood flow. Once the patient was safely with the paramedics, the policeman went to find the arm, which he retrieved from a shop doorway – when I saw the arm, it was in a Waitrose carrier bag. On a few occasions after a major incident, we have had riot or armed police on our unit after certain patients were admitted into our care.

Burglar, terrorist, a youngster high on spice, rapist, attacker ... We care for them, we don't judge and we treat everyone the same. It's best not to know their story, as they are all people and it often seems to me that some people have been treated the way they treat others.

Their back stories can be shocking. Father and son attack as a team. A mother's dominance and abuse leads to her son controlling and humiliating women. A gang of youths murder someone from another gang, possibly because he was on the wrong territory. So very often a person's upbringing and background directly influence who they become.

It seems that there are good people and bad people. But good people can be bad and bad people can be good. Any human can be pushed to the limit. Some youngsters who may be under armed guard are vulnerable and their young life has often bypassed a secure, loving and happy home.

On one occasion we had an issue with an aggressive young woman who fell and badly hit her head after a heavy night out involving drugs and alcohol. She had fresh stitches on her face and head and a deep wound, and she was awaiting surgery. This woman kept trying to abscond. The police were brilliant. They were there for a different patient, but on numerous occasions during the morning they helped us secure this particular young woman, dodging her kicking and punching and safely getting her back into bed calmly and professionally.

FEBRUARY 2021

7 February

I am worried that the situation is going to become so severe that Intensive Care will be rationed to those most likely to recover, with some patients taken off ventilators to make way for patients with a better chance of survival. There is limited capacity, but we give everyone the best chance. The numbers have apparently slowed down but we are not noticing this yet.

A patient was transferred from another hospital and arrived before a bed was available. She was Covid-negative but needed our expertise following an accident, and the hospital she came from had no beds at all. We had to plug her portable ventilator and oxygen supply into vacant ports in the corridor. As staff passed, they had to squeeze past her and the Critical Care transfer team, waiting for a bed to be vacated by a patient well enough to step down to a regular ward.

All the wards are mixed up or mixed together. Covid and non-Covid patients are divided safely to stop transmission of the virus. I have no idea where the respiratory unit or surgical ward are now. When you muddle up wards, equipment and the tools required to nurse and support a patient are all in the wrong place. I have no idea where to go to borrow a piece of equipment anymore. We needed a Doppler ultrasound (a small device that uses high-frequency soundwaves to meas- ure the amount of blood flow through arteries and veins). It was quite a mission to track one down; it's usually borrowed from the maxillofacial or vascular ward.

There is bureaucracy overload. We have changed our haemofiltration system – in the middle of a pandemic. We need to be trained or learn on the hoof how to use a different machine. The principles are the same for CRRT (continuous renal replacement therapy), but the consumables are differ- ent. The hospital's contract with the current company has expired, so now we use a different machine.

I have brain ache. The timing is appalling. Only a Critical Care nurse knows how to set up and care for this machinery. I have known few consultants who understand how to use and programme the machine, despite knowing the rationale for use, prescribing the treatment and understanding the nuances of osmosis and diffusion.

There is a national shortage of tracheostomy tubes, particularly the most common, sizes 7 and 8. So if a tracheos- tomy is performed, the doctor can only use the sizes available, not the size that best suits the patient.

Covid patients who have had days of NIV (non-invasive ventilation) using a tight mask definitely seem to fair far worse; their age and lack of comorbidities are dwarfed into insignifi- cance. They need intubation far earlier. It is a balance of risk: not putting a patient on a ventilator too late; but not too soon, either. We assess blood oxygenation, chest X-ray, respiratory rate and how tired the patient is. We always adapt our treatment and medical decisions based on our experience and research.

'Is this Clapham Common or Blackheath Common?' asked a patient, after I had put a nasogastric tube up his nose. I feel great warmth for a patient who, in his confused state in this strange and curious environment, believes that he is sitting on a common somewhere in London.

The deep connection I have developed with many staff is incredible. Some of them will have a place in my heart for ever. The Greek nurse with the amazing hair won my heart today, watching her kindness and sensitivity with a demanding and challenging patient. This weird place and space have triggered so many emotions. I knew I was strong and this has toppled me, but I stand firm and team work, team connection, team spirit and the shared experience gets us through. We support each other, care for each other and love each other. PPE hugs are the best!

Many of our patients require a CT scan. We have to gather up transfer equipment, portable ventilator, suction and a monitor. The CT scanner will always be on a different floor, so a bed and all the oxygen cylinders and kit need to be manoeuvred into the lift. So many lines, tubes and drips – there is always an impossible tangle created, which is meticulously unravelled by the ICU nurse following the procedure.

We are at war. We cannot hear the distant boom of gunfire. This is an invisible war. There is no respite when it gets dark at night: the lights remain on and we keep going, wading through the rubble and ducking when we can, with nowhere to hide. In some moments it is overwhelming. In others it's just hard work, and sometimes we simply feel tired and numb. Perhaps for medical staff the scars from this war will persist, as the scars of the First and Second World War lingered on into the twenty-first century.

We continue to work with support nurses as our backup. A colleague likened it to asking the cabin crew to land a jumbo jet. Their help is invaluable and unhelpful at the same time. There is a lot of button-pressing and knob-turning in a Critical Care environment; incorrect manoeuvres can have disastrous consequences. I see unqualified, untrained staff under immense pressure to help us and acquire years of knowledge, experience and training condensed into a ten-minute teaching session. We would not expect a person to be fluent in Japanese after 20 minutes.

We use masses of electricity and oxygen. There is a continual fire risk in the areas that are not equipped to deal with such a power demand by the complex equipment plugged into the few sockets at the back of the bed. Sometimes the area plunges into darkness and, after a few seconds, there is a deafening sound of all the machines beeping, hissing and pinging their alarms as a familiar, nerve-wracking, deep boom vibrates the area when the back-up generator kicks in. Patient safety is always at the forefront, but in the current climate we just do our very best and patients in our care remain safe. On one occasion the Trust's Fire Safety Advisor came to one of the Covid areas to brief staff on the above situation and how we maintain safety at all costs within the physical environment that was our temporary Critical Care unit.

Apparently, the numbers have decreased. Let's wait and see and hope.

*　　*　　*

We desperately need more nurses. The recruitment team were shipped out, off site to somewhere in Epsom. This saves money and diminishes working relationships. This team are a brilliant crew who seamlessly complete the pre-employment checks for new staff. They are a necessary and important cog in the wheel of recruitment and staffing our hospital. They are flexible and tolerate my 'on the hoof' emails, and work brilliantly when I put out an advertisement out to recruit more nurses. This can only be done following discussion, budget assessment and authorisation, which can take only an hour or up to a few weeks; it all depends on the money available in the recruitment pot. How amazing it would be to have enough money to recruit and train all the nurses we need.

14 February, Valentine's Day

'How was your day?' people continue to ask.

Well, this was my day ...

Covid ICU, in a temporary area created on a regular ward. Day shift; 12.5 hours (ish).

I work in a pod with four patients. I am alone apart from a support nurse who is usually based on a surgical ward. Later in the morning a nurse from clinic comes to help too. She qualified nine months ago and is enthusiastic and keen to help. It is hot and we have to keep the windows shut.

All the patients look the same. Middle-aged white men who are slightly overweight and have high cholesterol, type 2 diabetes and hypertension. We will keep going, keep giving meticulous care as staffing allows, but I know these four men will likely die. Men with families, friends, a profession. Men who, not long ago, were living a normal life. Three of them are proned, each with his body turned face down, creating a mound in the bed covered with a white sheet. All are ventilated, one attached to a haemofiltration machine due to kidney failure.

Deep breath, my day begins.

I move silently, gowned in my blue PPE straitjacket. I allocate tasks to my helper as I go back and forth. Suctioning, monitoring, changing ventilator settings, taking arterial blood samples, aspirating and flushing tubes and drips, changing

syringes, changing fluid bags, manipulating, fixing, straighten-
ing, balancing, adjusting, cleaning, measuring, recording.

Two of the men are unstable. I go between them, remind-
ing myself who needs what and when, my mind whirring in a
heightened state to ensure I miss nothing. I write a list of
drugs and procedures required for each man and I tick the list
as each task is accomplished. My helper, my backup, my naive
saviour supports me. Doctors enter the pod to assess and
evaluate care, prescribe further care and medication for each
individual. I challenge one decision and am asked my opinion
on another. I know and trust the consultant in charge.

One of the men becomes more unstable. He is on 100 per
cent oxygen and his blood-oxygen level is plummeting. His
blood pressure is dropping, despite the high amounts of positive and negative inotropes (drugs to support cardiac function)
pumped into his Covid-ravaged body at micrograms per kilogram per minute. This man is dead. Machinery and medication
are keeping his heart pumping and his lungs breathing and his
kidneys excreting.

I called his wife and asked her to come in. These phone
calls are so hard; a mask stifles my voice. She arrives with her
daughter two hours later, while I am clinging on to her
husband's life so they can be with him as he dies. The consultant updates them and explains that, despite all the treatment,
her husband is dying. My heart breaks for this devastated
family. They sit by his bed dressed in PPE as he fades, the
equipment and drugs losing their battle. There are no words
that help. But I answer their questions and offer silent support

and comfort. My helper is upset; she is not used to death in such brutal circumstances.

We wash the body, remove all the drips and tubes, and wrap him for the porters to collect and take him to the mortuary. The relevant Covid paperwork is completed.

Now I have three patients, but we clean and prepare the now-empty bed area for a new admission. We de-prone the remaining two proned patients (this procedure takes six members of staff). We turn the other man, adjusting his position to relieve his pressure areas. Many of the patients have pressure sores to their face or feet or sacrum (the base of the spine).

There is a hiatus. While another Critical Care nurse minds my patients, I grab a coffee and some cake, empty my bladder and chat to a colleague. It's a relief to be free of PPE, though I am cold, as my scrubs are wet from sweat.

The cardiologist arrives to assess one patient and perform an echocardiogram. One patient needs a new drip inserted into his jugular. Another is restless and needs a wash after opening his bowels. I take blood, insert a cannula, run a new CRRT filter circuit through for a patient whose electrolytes are deranged. Then I draw up syringes full of various medications delivered in precise amounts by a syringe driver.

The day flies by and I don't stop. I set up a new monitor, manoeuvre equipment, change haemofiltration fluid in five-litre bags that are so heavy, and the full bags of effluent need to be tipped down the toilet (our makeshift sluice within our pod) while avoiding 'splash back'. I look up blood results on the computer, change expired tubing, clean the men's teeth and wash their faces, carefully wiping around their tubes and pressure sores.

My helper fetches and carries and cries. She is learning fast. She collects blood from the blood bank and drugs from the pharmacy, so I am alone for a while. It is silent and still, except for the familiar hiss of the ventilator and a dull hum of so much electricity in action. Moments later, a patient's adrenaline pump starts screaming – informing me it will be empty in five minutes and giving me time to seamlessly switch to the next pre-loaded, life-sustaining syringe.

We check and administer the blood. One patient who is hypothermic (low body temperature) requires warming. There is a machine like a huge hair dryer that blows hot air into a special blanket to increase the body temperature. This man is septic, his body cannot control his temperature.

In Critical Care, as far as is possible, we normalise what we can to set parameters. All in an effort to increase recovery and improve survival chance. I give prescribed medication and the physiotherapist arrives to assess each man's respiratory function and requirements, offering chest physio to reduce secretions and improve oxygenation. The dietitian checks each patient's nasogastric feed to ensure they receive an individualised balance of protein and electrolytes – the feed dose is calculated by patient's weight and required calories. In critical illness, calorie consumption is massive, as the metabolic process is accelerated.

Many tasks need repeating every few hours. We record everything on a huge chart ... but where is my black pen? I start the day with three pens and often end the day with none. I might find one on the floor under a machine while another is accidentally stolen by another member of staff.

The new admission arrives, transferred from another hospital. Another Covid-riddled individual who we will try to fix. It takes us a while to transfer her onto our ventilator and pumps. I attach her ECG (electrocardiogram) leads to the monitor and untangle her lines. I suction her endotracheal tube. I ask our ward clerk to put her iPhone and glasses in the safe and upload her details on to our system to admit her into our care. I send my helper to find two extra pumps, as we do not have enough for the intravenous medication required.

We have a late lunch. Sometimes it's difficult to leave, as we are never quite up to date with tasks and procedures. I update my cover nurse, who is also my friend, so we chat about her new niece back home in Portugal.

I eat, but always too fast at work, as my body is set at a particular pace. Again, it's a relief to be PPE-free. I drink a bottle of water and return to find many doctors around one bed in my pod. The patient's heart is in an abnormal rhythm that is compromising his blood pressure and needs immediate correction using medication. I perform an ECG. I administer potassium, magnesium and calcium.

These patients are on a cliff edge. Covid dismantles them. We fight back and sometimes we win. Heart rate and rhythm corrected, the doctors leave – a junior doctor later returns with my pen. We reposition the patients, turn the heads of the proned, and once again there is calm in this pod of four silent mounds, machinery and equipment.

A team arrives to take the new patient for a CT scan. It is suspected that she has pulmonary emboli (blood clots in her lungs). Once again, lines become tangled as monitors and ventilator are transferred, along with portable suction, back-up oxygen and emergency drugs. I update records, prepare more medication and talk with a relative on the phone.

I am relieved when, at the end of my shift, a young Italian nurse grabs me from behind, hugs me and says, 'Boo!' She defibrillates my tired body back into life, her shining eyes looking fresh for the night shift. I relay the events of the day thoroughly and systematically. Then together we go through the monitor and ventilator settings for each patient.

I hug her. I hug my support nurse. And I leave the pod (finally, after returning twice to share further information).

'Go home,' my friend says.

So when you ask me, 'How's work?' This is how work was today. The next shift I am on is non-Covid ICU, so it will be entirely different.

20 February

Some days I think that I can't possibly keep going, and then I do. Some nurses are entirely broken. Some have already left, and some will never recover from what they have experienced. Many of us are strong, resilient and committed, though we will carry our battle scars for life.

We have an unequivocal moral obligation to treat patients, irrespective of any risk to ourselves. This is what we do, no question. We care for people who are stripped down to their bare human self. We are strong but diminished; we rise up each day to repeatedly face the monster.

Valentine's Day brought fabulous treat bags for the staff who were working. Red hearts and ribbons, donated by our ever-faithful and wonderful community, brought smiles to faces damaged from masks. These small things make a difference.

There are two empty beds. I dare not make a comment, as soon they may be occupied by Covid victims. Now it is not just Covid that takes our patients to the edge. There seems to be an increase in self-harm, and for an individual who is diagnosed as Covid-positive – this may be the last straw, despite being asymptomatic.

People are petrified about how they may be affected, their mental health causing mayhem, so they harm themselves in an effort to end their life and escape. We see those who do not succeed in committing suicide, but who change their lives for ever with the damage they cause to their body.

I once nursed a man who had made every effort to end his life. He planned it, accumulated the drugs and alcohol he would take, and then waited for his wife and children to be away for the weekend. It was a random visit to his home by a neighbour that saved his life.

When he came to in hospital he was devastated that his plans had been thwarted. He explained that it wasn't that he wanted to die or put his family through misery. He had felt as if he was on a carousel that was going faster and faster and faster, and he just had to jump off. He now believed he had been given a second chance and would do all he could (with support) to slow down the merry-go-round so he could climb off by himself.

If a person is without oxygen for a period of time because they are not breathing and their heart is not beating, then resuscitation commences. Some recover fully over time, but many do not. They are left with hypoxic brain damage (permanent damage caused by a lack of oxygen to the brain). These patients are stuck somewhere between life and death, often labelled a 'cabbage' by the non-medical.

Some who are brain dead will donate their organs, some people die and some require 24-hour care for the rest of their lives. It all depends on the circumstances of the event, and it is totally unpredictable who may or may not recover.

We keep temporarily running out of equipment or drugs, and then someone magical finds a replacement or adapts an alternative. We are ingenious and practical. We improvise, adjust and find a way, navigating the impossible.

Families can be hard work, each thinking they are the only one who has a relative who is denied visitors. The lockdown rules do not apply to them. I spend much time having circular conversations on the phone to a next of kin who thinks that the medical staff are being awkward or diffi-cult when we reiterate, yet again, that there is no visiting allowed unless a patient is at the end of their life. We don't want to restrict people who love each other being together, but this virus must be stopped. Therefore no visitors are allowed.

One of the best things I remember doing at work was bringing a patient down from the ward on her bed so she could lie next to her husband in his Critical Care bed. Both were 70 years old and badly injured when a lorry hit their car, and their beds were side by side for a short while and they held hands. Both recovered well.

It is supposition to say numbers are decreasing. The two empty beds are now full. In fact, as I write there is not one empty Critical Care bed. The reduction in Covid-positive individuals is not yet reflected in our actuality.

27 February

Critical Care nurses come from all over the world but we all speak the same language. I adjusted a patient's head and noticed that the pillow was blood-stained, thanks to a trickle of blood from a recently placed tube in the patient's neck vein. I was holding his head up, I pulled the soiled pillow out and, glancing at my colleague who without hesitation grabbed a fresh pillow from the end of the bed, I tossed her the dirty one and caught the clean one a second later. No words were spoken but a conversation was happening: the unique and slick exchange of understanding and pillows as we connected in that second. Colleagues, friends, ICU nurses, family – as

Critical Care nurses we know the urgency of meticulous attention to detail.

The volume of patients is astonishing. It's industrial-scale intensive care. I don't recognise this as my workplace. It's like coming home to find people have moved your furniture around and another family is living in your house. You want to get out, but the need to stay is strong, to ensure your home is safe and OK. The new family is lovely but they don't know where you keep the jam or the oven gloves or the vacuum cleaner.

Some patients are a diagnostic mystery. A patient collapses and is admitted to intensive care, but we have no idea what the precipitating factor is. Often we deal with the results of lifestyle choice. Alcohol and substance misuse cause liver failure. Years of smoking causes pulmonary disease. Reckless behaviour can cause accidents.

Various variants, surge capacity. It's like one long and protracted major incident. An ICU nurse is responsible for, and has to care for, double or treble their usual workload while supporting, teaching, explaining, guiding and working with a frequently changing support group. We work well out of our comfort zone, and I turn in ever-decreasing circles trying to give the best care, the best support, the best of everything I can. The pandemic diet of flapjacks and cake supports our calorie requirements.

The duration of this global Covid-19 pandemic and the extent of the devastation is uncertain, but repeatedly I hear that 'it's getting better'. There is now a plateau. Slowly we are noticing a change. We have closed one area but nurses are scared to relax – it ends when it ends and, for some of us, when it slows down we have time to reflect and think, and this is not a great place to be either. More tears happen and we are painfully aware that emotions are just below the surface.

Patients who I thought would die are recovering, through brilliance and persistence. We are incredible and very tired warriors who, despite everything, remain resilient.

The support nurses are amazing. One nurse said to me, 'I'm in a perpetual state of anxiety. Critical Care is so far removed from my normal job.' These nurses are away from their usual place of work, meaning their usual services are suspended. A haematology nurse, an oncology nurse, nurses from theatre, paediatric unit, day surgery, rehabilitation units, dementia services. Physios and speech and language specialists are helping in a non-medical capacity. Stocking up, cleaning equipment and helping turn and move patients. They empty catheter bags and suction canisters. Far removed from delivering chemotherapy, assisting a surgeon in theatre, supporting sick children and their families. We have all been shuffled like a pack of cards and dealt a random place to help during the pandemic.

After a tough day, two young nurses had back pain. We are trained to lift and roll patients using correct techniques to prevent damage or injury to staff or patient, but in a pandemic, with double or treble the workload, our backs ache. I rubbed the two young nurses' backs simultaneously.

It's good to care for each other. They are both young and beautiful, so I teased them and said, 'I am old and my back is fine.'

But they laughed and said, 'You don't work as hard as we do.' Always cheeky, always fabulous.

A man collapsed and was found by the police. A neighbour had noticed that there was a build-up of milk bottles on his doorstep and his curtains remained closed, so she had called the police. A well-dressed elderly woman came to visit him. We had not been able to ascertain a next of kin and we had received no enquiries. She was the neighbour who alerted the police.

She gave her mobile number as a contact, gave her work number (she was a florist) and her email address. She promised to return to visit the following day. She would act as a contact until one was found. She didn't know him but lived next door to him. A kind gesture. She added when she left – she was running late for work – that she was 94!

We plod on. I dream of lying on a beach somewhere glorious, with the sun on my face. I am not sure any of us will be the same again. I wonder how it will feel when we look back. We still have many patients, so the reduction in numbers does not yet translate. We are still busy. Covid patients who improve and recover are with us for days on end. When we continue to close the makeshift ICU areas, and there are empty beds and fewer and fewer Covid patients, we may feel it's getting better. But not one medic that I have spoken to is convinced this will be over just yet.

Here's hoping there will be fresh shoots appearing through the soil, like after a massive bush fire. It's spring, the vaccine is available. Perhaps this is the beginning of the end.

MARCH 2021

6 March

The coronavirus has been with us for just over a year, and the biggest question now is: when can we get back to normal?

A hidden reality is that thousands are currently suffering from the terrible after-effects of coronavirus. We may treat and fix and mend, but patients can go on to suffer for weeks with the aftermath: chronic fatigue, diarrhoea, breathlessness. Thankfully, many make a full recovery, but nothing is predictable with this virus.

It is the tsunami that hit us twice. The second wave, as brutal as the first, has now left surf that hits at a lesser pace, with the odd wave that knocks us over into the sea. We get up again and again and wait and hope, but we are not convinced just yet. Mainly, I think, because we cannot do this again.

Rehabilitation is at the forefront of our care. It's not like in a film where the patient wakes up, tubes out and all is fine. Physiotherapists work daily with Critical Care patients to aid their recovery. Their input with respiratory support is invaluable, as it is with making a plan to wean a patient from the ventilator, which must be done gradually, with breaks for recovery and rest. Many ICU patients who have been venti-lated for days or weeks will have a tracheostomy and need to learn to breathe unaided again. Patients are often weak with muscle wasting after critical illness and need to learn to move and walk again. Just sitting on the edge of the bed can be monumentally exhausting and requires help from at least two people.

Those who are tube-fed need a speech and language expert who assesses whether patients are able to swallow safely without aspirating (inhaling food into the lungs). A breathing tube in their airway for days or weeks to aid breath-ing can cause issues that take time to resolve, while a patient returns to normal breathing, swallowing and talking.

I have been touched by messages, cards and emails from patients or families that I've previously cared for. They have insight into the environment and see how we work when times are normal. It's amazing that they are prompted to send their best wishes. Even now, some families write a card to say thank you, when in the current climate we don't feel we have offered our very best.

There is one patient I have cared for many times. Years of substance abuse triggered, she told me, by an abusive father and then a partner. We fix her. Support her breathing, manage her hepatic encephalopathy (unconsciousness caused by advanced liver disease), drain her ascites (abnormal build-up of fluid in the abdomen) and discharge her, knowing that, sadly, she will be back. This time her situation was compli-cated with Covid, and this time, very sadly, she died.

Most people who get Covid-19 have mild or moderate symptoms, such as coughing, a fever and shortness of breath. But some who catch it get severe pneumonia. Sometimes it grabs at an entire family. Other times only one member of a family of five will get sick and everyone else is fine. I nursed a woman who had called an ambulance for her husband who had been ill with Covid for a week. He was dead by the time the ambulance arrived 20 minutes later. One look at her and they knew she needed hospitalisation. She was intubated and ventilated within 15 minutes of arriving at hospital.

Some patients are admitted injured or unwell and Covid is an incidental finding; they have no symptoms at all. There are a few Covid patients who have diarrhoea and vomiting with no respiratory symptoms. We still do not really understand this virus. It remains so unpredictable.

It's not all gloomy. There are jokes and teasing and laughing. We are a team. We are stronger together. A vast amount of coffee, cake and chocolate is consumed. One nurse had us in stitches, as she had knotted the drawstring of her scrubs and was dancing and joggling and yelping outside the toilet, with three of us trying to release the knot and help her out of her scrubs before she wet herself. 'Quick,' she kept saying. 'Quick, quick, quick!' Finally free, she flew into the toilet, letting out exclamations of relief as she emptied her full bladder.

Before Covid-19 paralysed the world, Critical Care nursing was demanding. Looking back, it was highly shocking when Covid erupted. I remember being allocated to a newly opened

Covid ICU area. Tension filled the air. It was like entering a war zone, with staff in bizarre apparel moving around at an unnerving pace and intubated patients being pushed along the corridor. Boxes of kit awaiting a home and the bewildered, anxious faces of the nurses. The adrenaline rush was palpable. These images still haunt us. This area now functions as a normal ward. I was telling a senior colleague that I'd walked towards the door to the ward last week, and I'd felt my heart pound as anxiety grew within me. 'You get that too?' she said. Many of us do.

As numbers are reported to be reducing, the achievements of the vaccine are celebrated. And as we close areas we escalated into, we start to relax. Frequently, I am still being *told* that it is better.

Better than what? Better than last week or last month or last year? It's still awful and exhausting for those of us still here, still going strong and still waiting – and even before Covid we were often pushed to the edge. When proning a patient yesterday, it didn't feel better. For him, it was terrible.

And when 'it is better' we will catch up with the masses of delayed elective surgery, the trauma calls as people go out and about again, the self-harm, those presenting late with illness who were scared to come to hospital, or those coming in as the result of lifestyle choice and overenthusiastic celebrations.

We will just keep going with the next wave of whatever is thrown at us. It's what we do.

13 March

A young woman suffering from puerperal psychosis (severe postnatal depression) walked in front of a truck to end her life. Her baby was only four weeks old. Thankfully, the woman survived and she was admitted to Critical Care. She was in shock, bewildered and in pain. Her full breasts were pouring with milk as her daughter was being cared for by the woman's aunt.

She wanted to die. She had no history of mental illness, but the swirling hormones of pregnancy and childbirth had caused such anxiety and deep depression that she needed to escape her life. Her husband was devastated and I suggested he come in to see his wife and bring their daughter with him.

When they arrived, I tucked the beautiful, tiny, sleeping baby into the crook of my patient's arm. She was tormented by the juxtaposition of her desire to love and feed her daughter while feeling incompetent and a failure as a mother. She kissed the little head for a second and then pushed her child away. My patient said she wasn't worthy to be a mother. Guilt now added to her tumultuous emotions. She withdrew into a dark place, and for days she battled the urge to terminate herself. She fed her baby or we expressed her milk. Sometimes she wouldn't look at her tiny daughter. Other days she held her close and wept.

I encouraged and supported her breast feeding. I believed her daughter was the key to her recovery. Post-partum psychosis is complex and these women need the correct treatment, care, support, love and time to heal.

We continue to bend but not break. We do our hopeless best. There are some empty beds and we clapped out a patient after 57 days of being on ICU.

This week has been a tough one for staff, especially after learning about the 1 per cent pay rise, which has communicated the value, worth and appreciation for all we have done.

The PPE remains our suit of armour and our nemesis, and we know that we need to drink to avoid the headaches and dehydration. Our faces have toughened to the continual FFP3 mask wearing. This is our routine now, our new normal, wrapped in plastic and paper, but we have each other.

While this virus might take away our social contact, the human need for touch and togetherness means nurses are connected in an inexplicable, visceral way. You cannot lock-down the human spirit.

Beds begin to empty. Some of the long-term Covid patients recover or die, and we look to continue to reduce our escalation areas. The support workers slowly return to their usual place of work, some damaged, some relieved, and some who want to return and train to be a Critical Care nurse.

I bumped into an ex-patient from the first wave in the corridor. He remembered my name and recognised me from behind my mask. I remembered the day we told his wife and young daughter he would probably not survive Covid-19. It was at the beginning, when I thought it couldn't get any worse but then it did. He looked fantastic, was back at work and was just coming to hospital for an outpatient appointment. My eyes filled with tears. He is one of our survivors. He is the reason we do this. So that some people will return to living their lives.

Plans are underway, after the endless yet mandatory meetings, to continue to de-escalate Covid areas. And here we go again – dismantle our fortress, deep clean, sterilise, disinfect and deconstruct and, as we unravel the makeshift Critical Care units, so we allow our emotions to spill and hope this is it for ever. The atmosphere is cautious. People talk about a third wave and there is a fear of us drowning.

A patient who is slowly recovering from Covid and will soon be transferred to the ward, after being unstable and proned at one point, is now eating yoghurt and learning to hold his body upright. Our patients eat mainly ice cream and yoghurt when first extubated as they are an easy consistency to swallow. He told me he needs to go home and see his cat and get some sleep. 'It's like being at Piccadilly Circus here. And has anyone ever told you – you talk so loudly?'

There was a moment of silence, broken by raucous laughter from the three other nurses next to his bed. 'Ah,' he said. 'I see you have been told this before ...'

We need faith, hope, love and laughter, and to look forward to the spring and the promise of sunshine, cafes and hugging friends.

'Freedom is the oxygen of the soul.'

Moshe Dayan

20 March

This weekend, the final two Covid ICUs will merge as one. Fewer Covid patients need our care or are revealed to be Covid-positive after being admitted for other reasons. They need ICU care but not for Covid – yet.

This time last year is hard to recall. I see the images in my head, which take me back to the battlefield when it first began. Unspeakable memories. What a hideous and life-changing journey that has rattled me to the core. I know I am changed for ever. Despite everything, I remain strong, determined, unbreakable and resilient.

This has been an extraordinary time and journey. I have cried and laughed, loved and worked like never before. I look forward to life and touch, being with other people, and to lying on a beach somewhere fabulous and hot. Lying on a beach is the only time I can truly relax, unwind and let go.

Just before I started working in Critical Care, I went to the General ICU during my night shift to collect my rota. I saw a senior sister with a patient admitted with a variceal bleed (swollen veins in the oesophagus that burst when pressures in the portal venous system get too high due to liver failure). She had a large Yankauer suction catheter in each hand and they were vibrating due to the speed of bleeding and the pressure of the suction as she stood at the head of the bed, suctioning the blood that poured from this man's mouth. She was relaxed, cool and in control, as she was trained, skilled and experienced. Another two nurses were administering blood at speed into the patient's veins to replace the blood loss, and a doctor was preparing to insert a Sengstaken tube – which creates pressure directly on the bleeding point to halt its flow – all to keep this man alive. It was exciting and stimulating and incredible. Life on the front line. She was so calm, chatting to me about my shifts, with all the bleeding, amid such a scene that was happening simultaneously.

No amount of blood is more shocking than Covid-19. The extraordinary explosion last year when patients were admitted one after the other, melting in front of us from this terrible virus that was knocking people down at an incredible pace. It truly was a tsunami that we swam in, and then we waded through the debris. For all of us, it was the death that was the hardest thing to deal with.

Now most of our Covid patients are long-term; they have fought and won and are ambling through the recovery phase of rehabilitation. The first proper conversation you have with a person you have proned, fought for, suctioned, washed and prepared drugs for is monumental.

One man had been so sick and was in the early part of his recovery – he just stared blankly, saliva running from his mouth, his tracheostomy tubing attaching him to the ventilator, wires and lines recording his vital signs. No eye contact, no smile, no response. He had been with us for days, on a journey that repeatedly skirted death, and now he tells me that 'toffee yoghurt is an abomination'. He is craving his sister's cheese omelette with chilli jam! He told me the scar on his arm was from a dog bite when he was nine, and that when his daughter was a baby he thought he would die of exhaustion. I reminded him that his wife probably felt the same. Truly incredible to chat and laugh with someone who could easily have been one of the many Covid victims that ended his stay with us in a body bag.

This digital world has provided us with the tools to communicate with family via video calls. I miss the relatives, as now I realise that this is how we learn about who a patient is – 'he's always grumpy' or 'a very private woman' or 'always the life and soul'. At least we have a platform for patients and family to connect. Staff find ingenious ways to rig up an iPad in the correct position; yesterday elastic bands secured an iPad to a pendant light above the bed. One patient said, 'No video call. They just say the same stuff. It makes me feel bad.'

Support nurses are returning to their original jobs so their service can resume. A technician who makes bespoke prosthetic limbs needs to be back at work so people can walk again. A paediatric nurse needs to return to care for children who need chemotherapy. A nurse from the cardiology clinic needs to see her patients who require care, education and guidance following cardiac surgery. This mish-mash of skilled, displaced individuals need to return home.

Will there be a third wave? Will we be prepared? Will we do it again? We wait and see.

APRIL 2021

Easter Sunday, 4 April

Easter is very different from last year, when we were in our tsunami, the waves at their highest, and we were exhausted and crying and scared. The PPE was new and suffocating. I taped my phone to a drip pole so a family could be with their loved one as she died.

I saw the death of so many in one day. I remember that we took turns to do CPR on a patient whose family had been talking to him on FaceTime, trying in vain to resuscitate this young teacher, the tablet still connected and bouncing around the bed with our chest compressions. This must be an image in this family's mind that haunts them.

The hideous, the funny, the sad, the unbelievable. The weeks and weeks that took over our lives and tore at our souls. I reflect on this time as I aspirate 20 millilitres of sputum from the subglottic port on a tracheostomy tube (secretion drainage tube) – who would think any job included aspirating spit?

A support nurse who usually resides in the community as an OT (occupational therapist), and who works with children with Down's syndrome, was asked to get an 'octopus'. She found the triple lumen extension lead used for giving multiple intravenous drugs, but she told me she was a bit baffled. Her vision was of grilled octopus and a lemon slice on a plate, but she knew that could not be what a critical care nurse with a sick, unstable patient had requested.

The very best Portuguese nurse gives her patient a spoonful of caramel ice cream. He has eaten nothing for weeks. This is the unstable man who kept me so busy on Valentine's Day trying to die. Now the look on his face as he swallows is that of a man at the best five-star restaurant in the world, sampling a tasting menu. I said, 'Now close your eyes and imagine you are on a beach.'

We are down to 13 Covid-positive ICU patients. Those who remain are mostly on the slow recovery journey with an upward trajectory. Pods are closed, machinery cleaned and stacked in the corners of the borrowed spaces. There is an eerie quiet where not so long ago the air was filled with noise and tension. Our shifts are slow and steady within the Covid ICU, but back to the normal craziness on the regular Critical Care areas that have claimed back their homeland and speciality.

The nurses' version of a Rubik's Cube: tangled lines and tubes woven around bed spaces from the plethora of equipment connected to patients who were fitted into the jigsaw we created last year. Covid is unravelling, it seems, and we hold our breath, hoping this is it – and hoping, too, that we won't unravel.

The team pulled together in order to survive and carry this load. Now we move forward, our strong bonds intact, as we were the only ones who, despite the madness, had a connection with so many people, while others were locked down at home. We were able to laugh and hug and talk and be together.

We shared much open and honest conversation, and it was the kind of sharing that might not necessarily happen in a bar or pub. We shared at the bedside. We are lucky. In a weird way, Covid has enriched us.

11 April

'Mask!' a young man from security yells. The gatekeeper guarding this fortress, lest a person enters the hospital without a mask. I don the blue paper mask at his instruction, a gesture that has become habit now. The absurdity of his own mask being under his nose escapes him.

Covid patients now number only ten in our Critical Care. We are taking advantage of the calm environment, focusing on the rehabilitation of the remaining survivors – cutting toenails, shaving a beard off where one would not usually be. We are our patients' family. These people have not seen their loved ones for weeks or, in some cases, months. It is genuinely with love and compassion that we administer some of our care now the war is ending. We see fewer doctors as they disperse, but our nurses remain, still bolstered by support workers whose learning curve has been enormous, some inspired to apply for a permanent job as a Critical Care nurse, others desperate to return to their actual job, which is frequently a totally different role in the hospital or community.

Our patients deserve meticulous care by a fully trained ICU nurse, one who is qualified and skilled, or one learning by working alongside their official mentor. This last year it couldn't be this way and senior staff needed to be vigilant for unconscious incompetence. It's how each drug is constituted and delivered, how to programme and manipulate our machinery; it's recognising and averting deterioration in a sick person, the gut feeling that develops in time. The sixth sense a nurse develops within their individual speciality.

It's quite tricky changing the tapes that hold the endotracheal or tracheostomy tube in place, even with opposable thumbs. To be gentle with the patient yet replace the dressing often soaked in sputum and sometimes blood, re-tie fresh tape ensuring that the tube is held securely in place, causing no pressure damage to the patient's mouth and lips. A young Scottish woman helps me. She is always laughing and today is wearing her scrub hat with the purple thistles. She looks fabulous but says the FFP3 masks make her spotty. I tease her: 'Teens are always spotty.' She looks so fresh, young and lovely.

Self-harm seems to be a casualty of this pandemic. People's mental health has declined. Their lack of employment and social contact, as well as being locked down at home, have caused untold distress.

I cared for a young woman who was a secure, confident uni student, but being away from her friends and attending lectures at her prestigious university from her bed in south London was not the aim and ambition that motivated her during her A levels a few years previously. Her usually happy home was disrupted when her parents decided to separate, which resulted in her consuming boxes of tablets. 'I don't want to die,' she said. The moment she swallowed the pills she called her mum. This young woman will be OK, but many cause permanent and irreparable damage to themselves – and some will die.

It is tremendous to nurse a person from the edge of life, where their unavoidable death is presumed and then, against all odds, they survive because we are brilliant and the patient is brilliant, and every second of effort was worth it.

To then buy the same patient a bottle of Coke, as that is his current craving, and laugh with him as the bubbles go up his nose, is an emotion for me that has no name but I feel it to the core. The connection a nurse has with their patient can be incredible. It's a moment of love, built from the nurse–patient relationship. Even if years later we don't even remember their name.

Usually we have all the same ventilators. There may be one we are trialling or we have a transport ventilator. Mostly, however, they are all the same. These are the ones we trained on, understand and are familiar with. But a pandemic brings all sorts of random ventilators: Chinese ones and some on loan from various companies; at one point we were using ancient anaesthetic machines.

Most of them have a similar interface, and the technicians have a laminated instruction and trouble-shooting page to hang on the side of each ventilator – a 'quick user guide'. But at 2 a.m., when lights are low in an aim to simulate night time – and when you can't find the light switch anyway, as this is an unfamiliar ward and not an ICU – you resort to looking for a demo on YouTube.

We have strict rules about talking English in front of patients, but in private spaces the sing-song of Spanish, Portuguese, Italian, Lithuanian, Polish, Tamal and Urdu voices warms my heart. Between us, so many different languages are spoken and the nurses switch backwards and forwards between English, their mother tongue and whatever language they have learned, adapting to each other and the situation. I have even learnt how to pronounce beetroot in Italian and hungry in Tagalog, the standard national language of the Philippines. And I love the Spanish phrase 'Madre mía', first heard when a bedpan of urine was slopped. These youngsters away from home create their own family. Brexit wants to exterminate them, and each week another one leaves and returns home to Europe. They feel unwelcome. We have lost 15 European nurses in the last six months. When they thank me for recruiting them and say that they have loved working at the hospital, I say, 'One day we will go out to lunch ...' in Milan or Lisbon or Madrid or Barcelona or Tuscany or Naples or Kraków or Athens or Helsinki or Porto or Bucharest or Budapest or Berlin ...

Never in Paris, though. In all my nursing career, I have never worked with or recruited a French nurse. Perhaps they're happy to stay in France.

We are vaccinated now. It is incredible that this virus did not catch us. Is the PPE that brilliant? Are we healthy? Are we immune or are we just very, very lucky? We continue to wear our 'suit of armour' but will not miss it one bit when the Covid door slams shut for ever.

18 April

Our main makeshift, temporary ICU has closed. The last patient left on Thursday. It is weird walking through a space that dominated our lives – twice.

Now being cleaned and sterilised, devoid of patients and alarming machines. Redundant chaos. It is silent and still. Just the pumps, monitors, beds and general clutter remain as the deep-clean team do their thing.

Again, we close for Covid business. The few remaining Covid patients take up side rooms in our regular ICU. They are recovering and rehabilitating. It is difficult to stem the tears, as this space has so many memories that only our team under-stand. So much death and so many survivors. So much compassion and resilience.

We are not angels. We are healthcare professionals who did our best to navigate the storm. Bruised yet still smiling, we now wait to hear where we work today. Though still rearranged to cover different areas, most ICU nurses are back home in their regular Critical Care, and our support nurses have returned to their own wards and depart-ments.

No one has escaped the effects of the pandemic. All of us, in some way, have been damaged. Lockdown is easing. Despite the cold weather, people sit together outside the pub drinking, laughing, chatting and hopefully healing – so good to see. The mood is lifting at last and will hopefully give some comfort to those who are still struggling.

Magic FM – or Covid FM as it became known – was the music of choice played in the pods. The fabulous and loved-by-all little blue radios donated by Empire Heroes Fund drowned out the electronic sounds, bleeps and alarms made by all the machinery and gave us a piece of normal. Now the radios lie in a redundant pile, waiting to be cleaned. Batteries spilling out where the back has fallen off and is lost somewhere in the detritus and rubble of the Covid aftermath. They, like us, need to heal, repair and stand up, to be ready to fill our days with music again.

*　　*　　*

It is the second Ramadan of the pandemic. Ramadan is a time for reflection, contemplation and celebration, a sacred time to worship Allah. Ramadan is on a different date each year, as its timing is based on the lunar cycle. Some of our Muslim staff are fasting, unable to eat or drink during daylight hours, and their prayers take on an added significance during this time, so a moment to pray during their long shifts in full PPE is important and necessary.

The hospital provides a prayer room but there is not the

time to visit. One of our nurses prefers to work night shifts when fasting, and uses the changing room as a place to pray. She tells me she clears her mind and then she can pray.

At the end of Ramadan, Muslims will celebrate Eid al-Fitr and the staff return to work. I see the henna stains from the artwork on the hands of our female Muslim nurses.

MAY 2021

1 May

On Wednesday a man refused a feeding tube. He was scared and anxious about catching Covid and had recently bought some geranium seedlings that he knew his wife would forget to water.

He had no appetite and his frail body needed sustenance. I chatted with him and explained why the tube was important; I understood his fear. I told him that I had inserted these tubes a thousand times, as I had worked on ICU for over two decades. I was quick and gentle. We discussed a process together and he allowed me to insert the tube and he was fine. A new Portuguese nurse helped and she could not have been more gentle. She was competent enough to insert the tube herself, but together we carried out the medical procedure in a slick, gentle and calm manner.

There is always a balance of sensitivity required with patients and family. To be kind, firm and help them feel secure and trust in our care. Communication with family is a learned skill that many nurses have and continue to develop throughout their nursing career. Empathy and humour are a necessary part of nursing. Some of our consultants in particular are superb at talking with family, showing sensitivity and kindness while clarifying and explaining facts about a loved one's condition and progression. Sometimes they explain that there is nothing more that we can offer, and help a family realise that we need to switch our focus of care to allow an individual a good death.

There is only one Covid patient on ICU, tucked away in a side room on one of our Critical Care units. That patient is recovering and, once fit for discharge, will be transferred to a ward. Hopefully that will be it – for as long as possible, but possibly not for ever.

Nurses are still bruised. I show them some artwork painted by Markus Vater. It is a large painting of the scene that swims in my head of the worst days of Covid. I described to Markus what it was like working in a tsunami and the tension, sadness, death and colour. Then he captured the images in my brain so perfectly.

I have a photo of this picture, and when the nurses see our memory committed to canvas it always provokes a reaction of sadness, shock and amazement. It brings back so many memories, and the eyes of several nurses and junior doctors have filled with tears on showing them the image. In full colour, it is the image that is for ever imprinted on our hearts and minds.

Sometimes we have the different victims of a single accident. Sometimes they are family or friends, or people from a different vehicle in a road traffic collision. We maintain confidentiality to protect each individual. Families are upset and sometimes devastated, blaming the other driver or alcohol, or an animal running into the road. There seems to be a need to apportion blame. But sometimes it's just an accident.

Nurses are quite crazy. Three of us discussed the different spices used in India to flavour the food in specific regions, and the heat and different flavours of curry in north and south India. Our new recruit from India shared her love of cooking and knowledge of spice learned from her mother-in-law. This conversation was had while we were filling a clinical waste bag with the cloths and pads from cleaning a patient. Is it only nurses who talk of food while the aroma of faeces fills the air?

It's good to go out again. To dress up and wear make-up, and to sip Aperol spritz in a balloon glass with ice. But it's chilly and I can't wait to have my Aperol served to me indoors or, even better, at the beach bar ...

At the end of the shift on Wednesday, I said goodnight to the man I inserted the nasogastric tube into. He squeezed my hand and said, 'Twenty-three years, eh? Thank you for twenty-three years of nursing.'

2 May

A piece of normal is so good. Staff are coming home to their usual unit and we are almost back to our regular one-to-one staff-to-patient ratio, which is safer. I am asked all the time if

I think there will be another surge. I have no idea. I didn't think it would happen a first time, let alone a second. I just appreciate us all being back together, our regular ICU family.

Our new staff bravely applied for a job not knowing if they would be heading for the storm or not. We hope to provide our usual support and guidance rather than drop them in at the deep end.

A family liaison team was created during the pandemic. They are a team of healthcare professionals from other areas and departments, and they communicate with and update family who have been unable to visit because of Covid restrictions, when communication between patient and family was only possible using FaceTime. When a family is at the bedside we update them and answer their questions. We learn about our patients, their likes and dislikes. A patient's personality is revealed through talking to family and friends.

Nurses need to individualise patients. During Covid, we had several patients each, who often looked similar: all had Covid pneumonitis, were on the same medication and were attached to identical machines and pumps. To humanise our patients we need to know who they are. A photo of a young man in cycle Lycra on a bike, or a woman with her dog on her lap, creates a dimension, a personality. Photos of family and pictures drawn by a neighbour's child all create a story of our patient; we learn about them, who they are, what makes them tick.

Usually the chatter from visitors at the bedside also reveals the personality and characteristics, and not always in a good way. Sometimes it is evident how little a family knows an individual. I remember a mum being astonished to see so many tattoos on her young daughter's arms and back. For some families this is how they learn their son is gay, as his long-term male partner is his next of kin. A man was admitted after collapsing during a marathon. 'I didn't realise he likes to run,' his father said.

This crisis and emergency situation can sometimes reunite a family – or not. If this is how a woman discovers her husband has another wife and child, it only serves to add to the devastation and shock.

We afford all our patients the same respect and offer the same expert care, whether they are an inmate from one of Her Majesty's prisons, a lord, a celebrity, a teenage mum, a teacher, a pianist, a famous actor, a doctor, a drug dealer, a person with dementia or a disability, a refugee, a sports personality, a transvestite, a member of staff. It doesn't matter who someone is or what they have done in life. We offer them our best care.

Sometimes we learn fascinating or hideous facts about our patients – but no matter. Each person is treated with kindness and given the best care possible regardless of their history. Colour, race, gender, age, sexuality, religion are irrelevant – these are our patients. Vulnerable, sick or injured, we are all the same: a human being in need of care.

At the beginning of the pandemic, our Head of Clinical Engineering planned and directed a 37-bed Intensive Care Unit in eight hours. These extra spaces were created and dismantled twice. Beds, ventilators, syringe drivers and smart pumps, monitors – so much kit, so many wires. Each bed area requires an oxygen and air port in the wall. Suction, plug sockets and space to fit everything – not easy in a space dedicated to a different speciality. Two regular ICU units functioned as Covid ICU, but the rest of the areas were temporary and often far from ideal, though we adapted and went with the plan.

A long-term patient's jejunostomy feeding tube (a soft tube that bypasses the stomach) blocked. Some of the medication we crush and dissolve makes a paste that we dilute in water and syringe down the tube. Despite flushing with water, these narrow tubes can block. It took five of us, including a dietitian, to get it working. We used all the recommended procedures, splattered the patient with Coca-Cola and hot-water flush, and once we worked out that the tiny plastic connection was the offending blocked piece, we were then ingenious in creating another connector: we joined two pieces of plastic from other tubes and connectors to finally create a functioning, non-leaking tube, thus preventing the need for the patient to have a new one inserted. He was unable to speak due to his ventilation method, so he wrote on a piece of paper: 'What happens if this fails?'

'Oh, we definitely euthanise you,' I said.

He laughed so much that he had a coughing fit. There is a balance, a connection, a relationship that is monumental and can be created within seconds. Nurse and patient. Trust, empathy and humour. From instinct and sensitivity, nurses can gauge appropriate and agreeable communication. With another patient I might have said, 'Don't worry, we will try to fix this. And if we can't we will insert another tube.'

With this man, my response was appropriate. We all laughed together, and he squeezed my hand so tightly, raised his eyes and shrugged his shoulders.

*   *   *

'Anthea! Stop running!' a teacher called after me while I was running down the corridor at school. 'No running in the corridor. That's why we have a playground.'

I was never very good at rules if they seemed silly, but I was well-behaved and respectful, so I walked. I wasn't in a hurry, but why walk when you can run?

When I ran the London Marathon, my first marathon (each marathon has been my last marathon, then I run another one), it took me to another level. I was proud of what my body could achieve, the strength and resilience I gained with this achievement. Less than 2 per cent of people run a marathon and one of them was me.

There was a moment, while running over Tower Bridge, when the crowds were cheering me – at this point there were only a few runners around me. My name was on my top. 'Come on, Anthea!' This powered me on, and for a moment I felt like an athlete, running over one of the most famous bridges in the world.

I liken it to having a baby. Months of preparation, eating the right food, not drinking, and reading tips on the final event. It was all in the meticulous detail and planning.

On the day, every emotion is experienced, from fear to elation. It pushes your body beyond its limits. It's long and painful, but the final push and cheering get you across the finish line and that feeling, that euphoria, is like when you are handed your newborn and you are seeing them for the first time.

And afterwards, it's the same as after giving birth. You decide never, ever again, and then your body and heart somehow trick you into thinking it's a good idea, and you should do it all over again.

Running is my alone time. I listen to Audible books or music. I make the best decisions while running and it helps me realign my soul. People often say, 'I saw you out running.' I don't see them. I am in my zone.

Working through the pandemic evoked some of the same feelings. Exhilaration came from success, teamwork and doing the very best we could do. Those special moments with our patients, the connection with colleagues. I knew I was strong, in body, mind and soul. I was ready to embrace the challenge and scoop up and support floundering nurses along the way. I worked with the most phenomenal group of human beings to care for those afflicted with Covid in the best way we could. My senior colleagues who ran the day to day were inspirational, and teamwork was taken to another level.

What an experience both were – running my first marathon and working through Covid. Both left me with the same feeling: Will I do this again? If I do, I know that I can.

9 May

CPAP stands for continuous positive airway pressure. This was the ventilation method used to treat many patients with Covid pneumonitis. I explain to new staff that it's like sticking your head out of a car window when it's driving at speed. It's a constant level of pressure greater than atmospheric pressure applied continuously to the upper airways. This can be administered via a tight-fitting mask or an endotracheal tube.

During Covid times anything thought to improve a patient's oxygenation was carried out to assist those with respiratory failure and deteriorating arterial blood gases. Often we proned patients and encouraged awake patients who were not ventilated to self-prone – to lie on their front for a period of time to improve oxygenation. Proning can improve ventilation and perfusion (circulation of blood through tissues).

Any method was employed if we thought it helped. It didn't always work but sometimes it made a massive difference. There were occasions when it was a last-ditch attempt to help a failing patient. A massive procedure for someone on the brink of life, but it gave them a chance and some of those patients survived and made a full recovery.

We see a fair amount of gang-related violence; it comes in waves. My friends in the Emergency Department update me on the fatal attacks, or the ones where the patient experiences minor injury. Beautiful young bodies attacked in such a brutal and senseless way, devastating the family and sometimes causing long-term, life-changing injuries.

I once comforted a young woman who was crying as her teenage son was dying following a knife attack. She was a young mum. Rather than being at home administering a curfew or buying him new trainers for football – his passion – she was asked to consider organ donation as brain-stem testing confirmed that his brain had died.

An impossible emotion for someone to process. Our brilliant team of specialist nurses for organ donation (SNODs) calmly explained organ donation as an option, and discussed if this was something her son would have agreed to. They explained the process without coercion or pressure, in such a kind yet professional way. After talking with her mother and sisters, she agreed. Her heart was broken but she knew that something amazing would come out of such a hideous situation. Her son was healthy and would donate his heart, lungs, kidneys, liver, small bowel, as well as skin and eyes. All to save or improve another person's life. Such a brave and tough decision.

I am always in awe of the SNOD team, who are so kind and gentle, and I am amazed at how a family can step away from their grief for one moment to agree to something so phenomenal.

I don't miss the battlefield medicine now. Our Covid patients are happily absent from Critical Care. The strength of our team has remained, and no one wants to discuss doing it again. We all say that we won't – but we will if we need to.

Confused patients send us all a bit nutty. A patient will often call out or say the same sentence repeatedly. During the night this is annoying and exhausting for staff, and it's a major issue for patients who are trying to sleep. It will not disturb our unconscious or sedated patients, but we have no idea if this noisy disruption affects them. During the day the shouting is diluted by the general hustle and bustle and noise that is Critical Care. 'Help! Get the police!' is a frequently heard phrase. More recently, 'I need to get to Asda. I need to go shopping ...'

One woman asked for driving directions. 'Excuse me, can you put the cabbages into the boot of my car? I grew them at the allotment.' One man needed to get to the pub.

Assume nothing in Critical Care.

Do not assume the Muslim woman wearing a hijab, when extubated, does not have a thick Scottish accent.

Do not assume the screaming from a non-English-speaking patient who cannot be calmed is fear and agitation, when after 30 minutes she gives birth to a baby.

Do not assume the woman who jumped off a building wasn't pushed.

A man in a suit may be wearing red lacy underwear. Another man may say his dog is his next of kin.

A young woman knocked over by a lorry had terrible issues with vomiting from the medication she was given. This is what we thought until a positive pregnancy test revealed the reason for her vomiting.

We accept and deal with what is in front of us. We always learn and we always do what we assess to be best practice with the known facts at our fingertips. One of our consultants would always say, 'When it comes to Critical Care – use this mantra and you will always be fine: Assume nothing, trust no one, give oxygen.'

8 May

A man had toothache. He had ignored his throbbing jaw and swollen cheek for weeks. Nurofen had numbed the pain, but when sepsis overwhelmed his body he collapsed and required an incision and drainage of a huge abscess in his neck. It occluded his airway and he had to be ventilated via a nasotracheal tube.

It took multiple people and the use of a GlideScope (a device used to visualise the larynx, which was swollen and bleeding), and to exchange the tube in his nose for a regular endotracheal tube. I held the nasal tube in position, and I was sandwiched between two doctors who were trying to insert a tube down his swollen throat. I was jammed at the head of the bed, between a ventilator and cardiac monitor. Another consultant issued instructions to support and guide the tube insertion. I angled my body to view the ventilator and monitor, so I could check the patient was stable and that he had adequate oxygenation during the procedure. Another nurse was administering drugs via a drip into the man's hand and a senior ICU nurse was passing saline flushes and various other equipment to the anaesthetist.

This is what happens. A squashed team of experts, behind the blue curtains, all focused on superb and safe care, early one Wednesday morning. This is solid-gold brilliance in action. Free at the point of care NHS fabulousness. During these moments I smile and say to myself, 'And what did you do at work today?'

Two days later, the man was discharged to the ward, drinking hot chocolate and eating rice pudding.

There is collateral damage from Covid. I don't think there is anyone who is unaffected. Mental-health issues amplified or new ones created through isolation and lack of social contact. I tolerate Zoom, as I have to, though really I need to see someone, interact face to face, touch them – the very things we now need to avoid. A friend leapt backwards instinctively as I moved towards her to hug.

As our world opens up for business again, I hope it will alleviate anxiety and loneliness for many. Bring back hugs and touch to release our oxytocin hormone. There's been too much self-harm. Too many people have attempted to or succeeded in ending their own lives. Too many people are scared, terrified to succumb to Covid's vicious bite.

Over 20 years ago an elderly man could not sleep. He was recovering from major surgery and was fed up. 'I just want to die,' he would say. I was working a night shift. The nurse in charge asked him how he got to sleep when he was at home. He told us that he didn't go to bed; he always slept in his chair. We padded up a chair, got him out of bed and made him comfortable. 'I need a drop of whisky, too,' he said.

After a team discussion, the pharmacist issued a measure of whisky. I was junior and had no idea this was even possible. My patient drank his whisky, slept in the chair and had a twinkle in his eye in the morning. Some things we do are so small but make a huge difference to the patient.

I popped into the cardiac intensive care to visit our one remaining Covid patient. 'Anthea!' he said when he saw me. This is the caramel ice-cream man who tried to die so many times. Now he couldn't be further from death. He is in the final stages of recovery, and he remembers our 'date' to one day go out for ice cream together. We don't usually see a patient out of work and this may never happen, but Covid broke barriers and rules.

The excellence continues, as does the hop, skip and jump to get things signed off and approved. There are many emails ccing managers and other managers and important Trust leaders whose job titles have lots of letters. The people in offices who are not Critical Care staff, who cannot possibly understand how it is on the shop floor but nevertheless make the final decisions, which have to be influenced by finances. Many meetings, many discussions. Apparently random decisions can seem short-sighted and not entirely appropriate. I see the angst of my immediate clinical leaders, matrons and head of nursing who do know what is required to run Critical Care, with or without Covid. The planning and execution are massive, and are what make our ICUs run day to day, week to week, year to year – patient care at the forefront.

15 May

Some people with Covid lose their sense of taste and smell. Some people have no symptoms at all. There are those with gastrointestinal issues or a headache or high temperature and, most common, those with respiratory symptoms. A continuous cough, which may lead to respiratory failure and high oxygen requirements.

Some patients are admitted with something entirely different and are found to be Covid-positive, and we have no idea if the two things are connected or not. I worked directly with Covid patients in Critical Care for months. I tested negative multiple times and have no antibodies. My neighbour who isolated at home, who adhered to the rules of lockdown and did not venture out of the house without PPE, caught Covid. Sometimes Covid would attack an entire family or only affect one person and no one else in the family, despite sharing a bed. Some people died from Covid-19 and some survived, and many died from complications related to the virus.

There is so much we still don't know or understand – the unseen enemy. I assumed at the beginning that I would succumb. Many of us did and we hoped we would survive. I was nervous about being a patient in my own unit or caring for a colleague. A few members of staff were admitted to Critical Care, but no one from the Critical Care team, thankfully, as I have no idea how I would have dealt with that crisis.

Something amazing happened during one night at the beginning of Covid, which I heard about in the morning. The bass guitarist Matthew Seligman, who had played with David Bowie at Live Aid, was a patient. Everything had been done to try to save him, but he was dying. One of our nurses played 'Heroes' at high volume. He died with nurses and to a song he'd played to the world during Live Aid, blasted out in a makeshift ICU in the middle of the night in Tooting.

The joy-pain-misery-triumph nirvana that I experience while running is often present for me at work: the contradicting emotions; the challenging thought process and instinctive and intuitive feelings that nurses experience. Nurses are the ones who are with the patients at all times. Doctors, physios and other healthcare professionals develop close bonds with some patients, but it is the nurses who spend hours and hours with patients and get to know them.

It is ideal when the team collaborates. The consultant will lead a ward round: a daily team discussion where each patient's care is planned and discussed, the results of procedures are examined and blood results noted, and medication is reviewed. Clinical examination of the patient is carried out and the consultant in charge for that day will discuss, document and share a plan of action for the day with the team.

This plan is reviewed and updated throughout the day, if and when required.

It's the nurses who often spot the tiny detail. The rash on someone's back, the contact lenses in the eyes, the forgotten HRT patch, the wound on the head. The nurses spend so much time with the family, so learn the detail. We develop close bonds, and during Covid this was hard for us.

A level of detachment is necessary in order to survive, but it is also important to develop a bond with a patient and their family too. It's a balance that can be challenging and it can take time to earn trust, yet we need to create a barrier to manage a professional and appropriate relationship. We just do this – from the heart and with instinct.

17 May

The Delta variant causes concern. My many Indian colleagues tell awful stories from their homeland of Covid and its effects on their community. India is in the midst of a crisis, with 4,000 people dying a day. We see the reports on the news and photos of patients sharing a hospital bed. There are concerns that the Indian variant could be more transmissible than the Kent variant, and there is a worry that the Indian variant could lead to a third wave.

At St George's the type of variant is somewhat irrelevant. If numbers do increase and we surge again, we need to deal with this once more. It's like a Ferris wheel that we keep jumping on and off.

This global issue is a conundrum that requires a solution. There are debates about vaccination programmes accelerating from twelve weeks to eight weeks for the second dose. Easing of restrictions may be in jeopardy if different variants cause a rise in cases.

It is paramount that we protect our NHS. I am not sure we can cope with a third wave of the tsunami, even just psychologically. Do we have the resources, the energy, the inclination? Our nurses are leaving. We are haemorrhaging senior staff, those who are trained and experienced. Mainly our incredible European nurses: Brexit topped with Covid followed by a 1 per cent pay rise and they are gone ... home to sunshine. Italy, Spain and Portugal. Our family is dispersing.

Perhaps the borders should have been closed sooner. I look forward to the day these questions are history and we reflect with dim, cloudy memory.

We have to be cautious about hugging. This is impossible for me. None of us realised a few years ago that one day we would be advised against hugging. Who could ever have predicted the events of the last 18 months? The next step of the road map may have a U-bend on it. We wait and see. Nothing is certain with Covid.

It seems that nurses, despite working in the same building, live in a parallel universe. During Covid it was horrendous, but even more so for the nurses on the wards who lost some of their permanent staff, as they were redeployed to support Critical Care. They had poorer-quality PPE and the nurse-to-patient ratio was far worse than on Critical Care. The outreach team saw the difference between Critical Care and the wards, which frequently were run by junior, inexperienced staff and student nurses who lacked the resources, expertise and equipment available in Critical Care.

Our matrons and senior sisters were adaptable, flexible, and sometimes they stayed overnight, trying to organise and plan. The senior non-clinical leaders working from home were not present – they couldn't be. Support came from within our team. Those who 'got it', as this is where they usually work. Clinical staff cannot work from home.

We had endless support from our community, in the form of food deliveries that we would often share with some of the wards: from CriticalNhs and the bakers from Earlsfield; from those who made scrub hats and dropped off treat bags for staff. From consultant to cleaner, our staff held up the world at St George's for a period in time, powered by the generosity of strangers, some of whom became my friends.

Usually a hospital is run from top to bottom. We all play a part, but the pandemic created a leadership from the inside out, run by those who working with Covid, on the shop floor. Those who were in the crisis, in the building, experiencing the reality, and the staff who supported the non-Covid patients and the regular functioning of a hospital. From Emergency Department to the wards, pharmacy, CT scan, outreach, X-ray, physiotherapist, microbiology, blood bank, theatres. dietetics. So many different people and departments. Our staff.

Today: Monday, 17 May 2021 – zero Covid patients on ICU at St George's Hospital.

Can we breathe now?

22 May

Those with lifestyle choices that colour their judgement sometimes flock together. They provide a mutual support system, not always healthy when based on substance misuse, but in some cases can lead to a happier ending.

There was a situation when a patient was admitted after having collapsed. We had no known next of kin. The police investigated and found out that a patient in a different unit was in fact the partner of our patient and was also lacking a known next of kin. A couple united through companionship, both attached to machinery, and days later we joined the dots.

A man came back to visit recently, bringing his daughter to the hospital for an appointment. Eight years ago his friend's car had skidded on the ice and hit a tree. He was in the back seat and, as his friend had recently deposited some old chairs at the council refuse site, the seatbelt had become wedged and was temporarily unusable. There were four of them in the car and they were going out for a drink. The driver had not been drinking. When they skidded, our patient was catapulted through the front windscreen, hitting a tree, then ricocheted backwards through the rear windscreen, landing several metres away. This caused his brain to collide at high velocity with the bony skull in which it is housed.

I was with the consultant and our patient's pregnant wife when the news was broken: he needed brain surgery and cardiac surgery, each causing potential risk to the other surgery. His wife was told he was unlikely to recover. He did recover, though – against all odds. Except he says he sometimes forgets things and he's gone off cooking, his previous passion, but otherwise he is fine.

I am tired. The struggle and survival have exhausted us. Standing at the bus stop in the rain, my knee painful as it makes its slow recovery from a torn meniscus. Negotiating umbrella, mask, bag, strapped knee and my phone as I pay my fare, tapping on the yellow circle as I board the bus. I need to rest and lie down in the sun.

Although we have no Covid patients, we are tired from the relentless battering. People say, as before, 'It's great – the numbers are down.' This is good, but sometimes the spirit weighs heavily and the knee throbs. We are still tired, still recovering.

Ears are great. We listen and we hear, if we are lucky enough not to have any hearing impairment. Ears became overloaded during Covid. I noticed one of our nurses on his way in to work, with glasses on, mask on, earphones in. His ears were busy. Later I saw him with a pen behind his ear.

One of our nurses is slightly deaf and she is always flinging her hearing aids through the air when she removes her mask, as they get caught in the elastic. Many times she would struggle to hear, as the masks muffled our voices and she could not rely on lip reading.

I am happy that nurses still seek me out for chats or hugs, or for advice or support. They often bring me an Americano from Pret without my asking. When I am office-based I leave the door open, and nurses pop in to say hello or chat and check up on me. I have so much time and affection for these nurses.

One nurse talked to me about an incident that had been bothering him. Once he explained, I could understand his anxiety and was able to reassure him. He bounced into the office yesterday to tell me the same situation happened again but this time he understood the circumstances and was able to deal with the problem. 'And would you like a coffee from Pret?' he asked.

Doctors diagnose and cure. Nurses treat and care. Together we unite, doing our absolute best.

Every day I work I get the same feeling. There is always someone who knows the answer – how to operate a piece of machinery or how to constitute a particular drug, where something is kept or how to book a transfer, how to set up skin traction or operate the breast-milk pump. The hospital policy for dealing with a particular situation, who signs a request form. How to get the curtains changed or obtain a certain piece of respiratory tubing.

We are a team, made up of consultants, matrons, doctors, nurses, physios, technicians, dietitians, students, housekeepers, healthcare assistants, practice education team, ward clerks, receptionists, pharmacists, cleaners, research and audit team, service and general managers. There is always someone who knows.

We are now back in our comfort zone and each one of us is hoping silently that we are done now, that this is over.

JUNE 2021

1 June

The UK has announced zero daily Covid deaths within 28 days of a positive test for the first time since March 2020. This is great but there is a new epidemic. Mental-health issues. Self-harm, especially among young people, some of whom have never experienced a mental-health problem before. Increased depressive and anxiety symptoms – the result of lockdown and living through the past year of unpredictability and fear, economic and educational stress, and without normal coping mechanisms.

I have spoken to friends, neighbours and colleagues. They all know of someone who is struggling. I hear stories of so many issues relating to anxiety and mental health in children and young adults. From low-level anxiety through to serious psychiatric illness. Some may already have had issues that were exacerbated by the pandemic.

Eating disorders, cutting and refusing to leave the house. A colleague told me her small son was scared at nursery, as he had never met other babies and children before. One of our consultants has taken time off to support her daughter, who has dropped out of university. A neighbour's son has been diagnosed with bulimia. Another young adult I know has anorexia, and a friend confided in me that her daughter is cutting herself. I know of two families where there has been the recent suicide of a teenager.

We need to support these individuals, help them find a non-destructive way of helping themselves, with community or in-patient support. We must recognise warning signs and nurture these people back to safety.

When a healthcare facility is alerted a risk assessment is performed by the psychiatric team, and sometimes it is necessary, for a person's safety, to detain them under the Mental Capacity Act (MCA). This is usually because someone is unable or unwilling to consent. Mostly with therapy, medication, time and caring, they will heal or manage their mental health in a more positive way.

We need a fresh perspective. The mantra of 'hands, face and space' and the slogans designed to help us now need to remind us to recognise that people may be struggling. The pandemic happened to us all. The wave dodged no one. We need some light relief and to feel safe, to touch each other and be together again. Masks block our facial expressions, communication and our kisses. People are scared of physical connection. They have not hugged anyone outside their immediate circle for months. Who knows if the go-ahead to ease restrictions on 21 June will be delayed. This will depend on a rise in cases of coronavirus.

Institutional knowledge of mental-health issues concerns

me. So many patients have tried to end their life. We see young and old patients whose attempt was unsuccessful, but who still may die or experience the long-term effects of a life-changing injury or organ damage. Overdose, hanging, jumping, self-inflicted wounds – all desperate measures for an individual to escape what is haunting them.

Nurses are leaving or cannot sleep, and many are seeking counselling and support. All staff were affected and live on a knife edge, waiting to see if we do this a third time. Unpredictability can cause insecurity. I have observed myself the sharp increase in the amount of mental-health related admissions to Critical Care.

I check our staff communication bulletin regularly to see if Covid admissions are rising. Once Critical Care reaches a magic pre-set figure, we climb aboard the Covid Express again and escalate into other areas.

Nurses bounce back from adversity – we are resilient. The abiding element is a sense of community. We are a family. We all need to accept the status quo and move forward and embrace the way things are now, but the aftershocks will last for years. Mental-health issues increasing, waiting lists are longer. We need to prioritise patients' surgery and be tolerant of the demands and irritation from patients who feel abandoned. I see queues outside the Emergency Department of those waiting to be seen by our tired, depleted team. Every day is busy. A lack of beds or staff shortages are dealt with with admirable efficiency and leadership. It's like a very complex game of musical chairs.

The vaccine-versus-virus race is underway. Single vaccine, double vax, still waiting, and the anti-vaccine group.

We need to keep on keeping on. We need to win in the race.

*   *   *

Sometimes my home and work life collide, as I've mentioned before. Living and working close by is bound to create a connection. There have been times when I nurse someone I know or recognise. I am a professional and respect confidentially and would never want a person to feel embarrassed or awkward.

One extraordinary situation was in November 2016, when I was called early in the morning and asked to attend an emergency meeting just before my shift was due to begin. I was in charge that day, and a major incident had been declared. A tram had derailed in Croydon and the hospital were expecting multiple admissions of severely injured people.

My son was 11 and went to school in Croydon. Usually he took the train and bus with friends, but on this day he went in early to look for a missing geography book.

I had been at work for two hours. We had a plan that was made with senior staff and our site manager. We were organising beds and staff, and were aware that most of our admissions would go from the Emergency Department to theatre and then to Critical Care.

My son called me. He was stuck, he told me. Following the accident with the tram there were emergency vehicles and police everywhere. He had ducked under the blue and white police tape, as this was his route to school, and now he was lost and didn't know what to do. He had become disoriented amidst the chaos. My son was spotted by a policeman who spoke to me on my son's phone and kindly directed him away from the situation and in the direction of his school. I then carried on with my day and we admitted several patients injured in the accident. Later, I learned that my son's school had opened its canteen to emergency staff so they were fed throughout the day.

11 June

Whenever a day was tough or something was bothering me, I would turn to Jonathan, my soulmate and confidant. I would bury my face in his tabby fur and listen to him purr. I have always had cats and I particularly love tabby cats. So six years ago, when I saw the expression on the face of an eight-week-old stripy kitten being held up for a photo on Gumtree, I knew he was the one. And he was. We drove to Maida Vale to collect this pot-bellied little purring ball of fluff. He smelt of curry.

He was spot on. One in a million, and a cat who loved me back. He would sit and wait for me when I came home from work. After the long, soul-destroying days during the pandemic, I would snuggle up with him and feel peace and warmth and love. Every night he would sleep next to me and press his face against mine for a kiss or stroke.

I loved him, and a piece of my heart broke when, a few days ago, he was run over and killed instantly outside our front door when someone in a grey Mercedes was in a rush. He was only six, and it happened the same day that I had knee surgery. When I was just beginning to return from the dark place Covid took me to, my beautiful cat was taken from me.

Do things happen for a reason? No. Life is random. Good times, bad times. I guess you need one to understand the other. I don't think things happen for a reason. I think life just happens, and it's how you deal with it that's important. For me, I cry (in fact, I wailed). I felt like my heart had been ripped out. I felt angry and why, why, why?

Jonathan, my beautiful cat, will always have a place in my heart. He had a fabulous life and some relief came from knowing he was killed instantly. I cry, I wallow, I remember, I question, I heal and I keep going, as this wasn't 'done' to me. It happened to me.

Accidents are what I see and understand. I care for so many people following an accident. I try to support and connect, as there are no words that bring comfort when your heart is broken.

The families of my patients try to find a reason and often there is none. One second later or earlier – would that have made a difference? To not have got in the car, stayed home, not taken that drug, not stood on that balcony, not crossed the road. Too late now.

We need someone to blame. There is often no one to blame. I remember trying to comfort a firefighter whose brother had been killed in a work-related accident. He was distraught and angry and desperately wanting to blame someone. A floor in a burning building gave way. It was an accident. This man had no place for his grief and emotion, his shock – the numb, hideous feeling of losing someone you love. This big burly man, in uniform, sat on the floor in a hospital corridor and sobbed. I too sat on the floor and put my arms around him.

Grief is painful, but the reason for grief is love, and that's what we need to hang on to.

14 June

Lockdown easing in England delayed until 19 July is announced today. The brakes are on in the escalation towards stage 4 of the government's 'roadmap'. The most severe cases of Covid are among unvaccinated people, or those who have only received one dose of the vaccine.

The effects are not yet being felt in the hospital but we are on alert. Trained and experienced Critical Care nurses continue to leave and so far have not been replaced. This will be my job once these positions are signed off by the various people who authorise and approve: the layers of management and finance departments who agree the spend on vital staff who keep this great ship above water.

Twenty-four band 6 nurses have left in the last seven months, since the autumn of 2020. Band 6 nurses are experienced and fully trained Critical Care nurses. Mostly they are 'home-grown' nurses we have invested in, educated and financed. Now they take their skills to a different establishment, as there is no opportunity for promotion because we are saving money and do not have the budget to offer them a financial incentive.

The European nurses are returning home; they are a massive loss for us. However, I am the lucky one, as these wonderful nurses still include me and come and eat Portuguese dough-nuts in my garden and call me via video from home or wherever they have travelled to. Last week I had two calls from nurses who have now left, just to say hello and see how I am. These surrogate daughters make my heart happy and I am so proud of them and their achievements. I get such a warm feeling knowing that I connected a group of strangers from many different countries and now they are friends for life.

A spreadsheet tells us how many staff are required and that's what we are funded for – no backup for those seconded to another area or those on sick leave, maternity leave or a career break. Spreadsheets have a different perspective on how the staff understand the situation.

New nurses have started but they are new to Critical Care and lack the skills and experience. However, they are training and learning to be competent ICU nurses. It costs more to recruit and train a new nurse than it does to promote an exist-ing nurse. I assume there is something I don't understand, or there is information I do not have. For me, from the shop floor, these decisions seem short-sighted and bonkers.

St George's has never been pushed like it was in the first wave of Covid. It was tested to the limit. Somehow the NHS finds a way. During the first wave, normal services stopped. The entire NHS stood down its elective programmes, as it was the safest thing to do. We focused on Covid. But during the second wave we continued to try to run the hospital. We were still recovering from the first wave while being hit by another. Like picking yourself up in the sea when one breaker hits, you stand back up, don't quite get your balance, and a larger breaker knocks you over again. No sea, no sun, no beach here, but definitely the taste of salt in your mouth.

The second time, we realised that we needed to keep going and come to terms with living like this. For the sick or injured patient, it's only the now that matters and we do all we can to treat and care. We integrate Covid into our lives and run our Critical Care as before. We have the skills, expertise, knowledge and experience.

Caring for the elderly is a massive part of our work. I am always in awe of the determination of some people who, despite being frail, retain a positive attitude. While living and working in Australia, I worked in many different nursing homes and met some fantastic people. I met a nun who had been a prostitute and a man who took up ballroom dancing in his eighties. Elderly people are fabulous, such fun and brilliant to work with. The odd one is grumpy, but we have grumpy young patients too.

Walking down Tooting high street in the rain, I see a young man cycling no-hands, holding an umbrella with one hand

and texting on his phone with the other. This man is at more risk of an accident than catching Covid. He would probably recover from Covid. His current actions could lead to life-changing injury or death. I see a recycling truck coming in the other direction. I wince. He wobbles as he cycles past the heavy vehicle and rides on.

21 June

I am so lucky. Today I spoke to one of my nurses, who is working in Aruba. She was just about to run a half-marathon at 4 a.m. 'It's too hot to run a race during the day,' she explained. I track her on the app she forwarded while I listen to Tina Turner and make biscuits. I look back over my diary entries and see that on this day last year I wrote: 'I love to run. I ran a half-marathon shortly before Covid took over my life and I am just back to running longer distances. Running clears my mind and it feels great to escape. It is my therapy and my time alone to recalibrate ...'

I spoke to another of my nurses, who is working in Sudan and was sitting by the pool. I watch the rain in Balham as she video calls from the heat in Africa.

JULY 2021

4 July

Death fascinates me. I think it fascinates many people but they wouldn't admit it. Death doesn't scare me but I'm certainly not ready for it – I would prefer to get my underwear drawer in order and travel more and spend as long as I can with the people I love. So no time soon, please.

I'm fiercely independent. There is life or death and I never want to be stuck halfway between the two camps. If I can't wipe my own bottom and you can't discuss this with me, then it's curtains.

I tell people that, as I live locally, I'll probably end up in the mortuary in St George's Hospital, but I always get looks of horror. My cousin was registrar at Highgate Cemetery for ten years, so perhaps our relaxed attitude to death is in our blood.

I would quite like my funeral before I die. The idea of all those I love in the same room at one time – I certainly wouldn't want to miss that. I tell my family that I want a big send-off and celebration of my life with Champagne and a chocolate fountain. One of the nurses I mentored when she was a student in Critical Care, and who is now a brilliant ICU nurse, always laughs when I say this, although I tell her that she will get to the mortuary faster than me. She wears a hijab and pins it to secure it in place. I see her wince in pain as she jabs the skin on her head with a tiny pin. She always loses the pins, so I bought her a coloured selection of pins for her birthday and now she sends me a photo of that day's pin colour against the black fabric. When they scan her brain, I tell her, it will be full of metal from the lost pins.

We do all we can to help a person survive injury and recover from illness. Every patient gets the best care we can offer, and when there is nothing else or a patient starts to fade, we ensure they have the best, most dignified death possible. Once an individual dies, it's as if they are totally gone. Their body remains but their soul, their personality, their individuality, their essence has climbed out and left. For this reason, I find the mortuary a calm place, devoid of atmosphere; not eerie or spooky or weird – just another space in this hospital.

As a student nurse, I spent a day working in the mortuary. I watched a post-mortem. The body was prepared by the anatomical pathology technologists (APT), who are trained and skilled. The organs were removed to be examined by the pathologist. Then the body was reconstructed afterwards. It was the most incredible way to learn about anatomy, and a surreal experience with Vicks VapoRub applied to the inside of my nose.

Badly damaged or dismembered bodies from trauma are repaired. These skilled and gentle technicians meticulously and carefully put a person back together, to make them whole again, not just for their loved ones but simply for the dignity of the individual.

In the basement at St George's there is a massive mortuary – a labyrinth of corridors to areas with fridges and freezers. Within each tall fridge and freezer there are five to six metal trays, and a trolley with an adaptable height is used to insert or remove a body. There are several post-mortem rooms, the largest of which has a viewing gallery. There are dedicated fridges and deep-freeze facilities for regular, high-risk and bariatric (obese) cadavers. There is a fridge for babies and foetuses, as well as shelves where specimens are stored, perfectly labelled and ordered.

St George's mortuary is one of the largest in the country, with space for 198 bodies. There are also temporary mortuary facilities since Covid. During the first wave bodies needed to be transferred to a temporary facility in north London due to the lack of space.

The mortuary's work includes routine coroner's post-mortems to establish cause of death, forensic post-mortems in the event of an unexplained death and high-risk post-mortems of infected patients, including those with Covid. The mortuary serves all of south London. If a person dies there is an option for corneal, tissue or joint donation, which takes place in the mortuary and requires hours to harvest by a specialist retrieval team. Some people choose to donate their body in its entirety to medical science.

The mortuary is clean and cool, with mopped tiled floors and large metal sinks. The fridges have each patient's name on and their date of death. Everything is ordered and meticulous.

Those who work in the mortuary do a phenomenal job, but as it is unseen it gets forgotten. And anyway, no one wants to think of death. At the height of the pandemic I went with one of our matrons to drop off boxes of biscuits and chocolates to say thank you, as they were so busy not only dealing with deaths within the hospital, but also from the local community and care homes. Those pronounced dead outside of hospital come directly to the mortuary. In one weekend at the height of the pandemic, Covid deaths, as well as the 'regular' deaths, totalled 88. The staff were under enormous pressure as coronavirus raged.

The staff have seen some horrendous and disturbing sights: decomposed bodies, or those severely damaged by trauma, or victims from a fire or attack. They might have seen multiple bodies from a terrorist attack or major incident.

Their work is complex, involving extended knowledge of the human body and how it functions. The staff are not squeamish, of course, and they deal with heartbroken relatives who come to view their loved ones. There is a large white cot in the corridor, donated by some bereaved parents, and it is for a dead baby or child to be viewed in. The staff pay attention to detail and recognise how important the little things mean to a family.

Bodies remain in the mortuary for a few days – longer for forensic cases or if a body's identity cannot be established. One body remained in the mortuary for 15 years. Once a body is released, it is collected by the undertaker and transferred in preparation for a funeral.

The body of every person who dies, regardless of age – from premature baby to someone who has passed their hundredth birthday – is always treated with the utmost compassion and respect. The mortuary is not a place of inherent sadness for those who work there, although the loss of an individual can cause total agony for those who love them. The mortuary is where we all go at the end of our life. It is a place where the staff are respectful and sensitive, and they feel privileged to work in their department.

*   *   *

At St George's we deal with the beginning of life. Tiny, perfect and healthy babies – and those not as fortunate. Some babies during pregnancy may require intervention. *Baby Surgeons: Delivering Miracles*, a Channel 4 series, followed the work of maternal-foetal medicine specialists at St George's operating on babies within the womb.

We deal with the end of life. We have a palliative care team, specialists who support patients at the end of their life who require symptom control and pain relief.

The Emergency Department is busy 24 hours a day all year, and since 2014 has been home to the Channel 4 series *24 Hours in A&E*. Patients following major trauma are admitted via the helipad, flown in by HEMS (helicopter emergency medical service), or via blue light in an ambulance. Staff in ED deal daily with everything from accidents and emergencies to those who come in with minor injuries, those who are inebriated or perhaps partied too hard, and many people who are suffering from acute mental-health issues.

St George's deals with complex and simple elective surgery, covering countless specialities. Our hospital is amazing because of the incredible and dedicated staff that work in this vast collection of buildings and Portakabins: the maze of departments, wards, clinics, theatres, laboratories, seminar rooms, simulation centre and much, much more. We support and care for those who need us, from delivery suite to the mortuary and everywhere else in between, within these many walls.

18 July

The day before lockdown rules end. Tomorrow is Freedom Day, as it has been called. All legal restrictions on social contact are to be removed. Our Prime Minister states that it is important to proceed with caution.

Freedom means you can still catch it and pass it on, but you can be out and about freely. Nightclubs will open, no limit on how many people can attend weddings or funerals, and those working from home will begin to return to work.

Some people wear a mask while alone in their car; others refuse to wear a mask. I see people in the supermarket with masks on and their glasses have steamed up. Now we have individual responsibility. Some people wear masks over their mouth only or under their chin or not at all. Masks are often a bit grubby, dug out from the bottom of a handbag or pocket, or are hung on a wrist or elbow. Some are worn upside down or inside out. Some wear FFP3 masks with diligence and determination, their battle armour to meet the headwind full on.

Tomorrow morning, Pret will remove all the Perspex screens and one-way signs. Personally, I find it refreshing to revert to the old ways. But many people prefer to wear their mask and keep their distance.

Outside the coffee shop in Balham, an orderly queue forms with a one-metre space between each person. We have 'long lockdown'. People find it difficult to step forward or step away. We have become conditioned to segregate ourselves from each other, and when meeting friends there will be a do-we-hug-or-not moment. I always defer to a hug.

Today, I arrive at work and am allocated to care for Covid patients in the 'blue zone'. Two days ago we flipped an ICU area to a 'blue area' for three Covid-positive patients. I don't understand the random Covid pathway colours the hospital uses to denote the level of severity. Super green (Covid-negative with 14 days of isolation), green (Covid-negative), yellow (Covid-negative but no isolation), amber (awaiting result), blue (Covid-positive). During the peak of the pandemic nurses decided that blue was the colour you turn when you cannot breathe – when you are hypoxic. This is not the reason blue is used, of course, but simply inappropriate nurse humour. Colours are used a lot.

Blue is the colour of Covid. There are many colours used to describe or explain something at work. Yellow for jaundice. Red is for blood. Code red – massive haemorrhage. And then there is brown ... Patients are prescribed laxatives because constipation can be an issue in hospital. Constipation causes pain, especially as a patient's mobility is limited and the diet is different. However, when a patient seems to be constipated or have diarrhoea, achieving the balance is a skill – and the phrase 'code brown' is understood by all nurses. Or 'brown code', as one of my Italian nurses calls it.

Some Covid patients who require Critical Care reside in side-rooms on our cardiac unit. We needed extra beds, so three patients were admitted to a bay on Brodie Ward. That's the ward where it all began in March 2020. I felt numb as I entered the space that once consumed us, where I first saw nurses struggling and was inspired to write my first email asking for support and biscuits.

The atmosphere is different now. The war zone has gone. This is just a five-bedded bay within a ward where the label printer still doesn't work and the cupboard door containing oxygen masks still swings open because the hinge is broken. The phone at the desk doesn't sit properly on its base – it wobbles. The staff toilet is a good size and the taps at the sink work well.

On this occasion, today, we care for two patients who chose not to be vaccinated. Some of the Covid-positive patients who didn't have the vaccine are now really sick, so sick that they are unaware of the consequences. Two of these patients have since died, and as they are dead I don't know if they changed their minds about the vaccine or not.

One patient was concerned about being controlled by the government, having a 5G chip injected into him. Some patients 'didn't get around' to being vaccinated. Some chose not to be vaccinated, as they didn't trust the research or they were worried it would make them infertile. I suppress my personal opinion. All our patients are given our very best, non-judgemental care. Some people choose not to be vaccinated because they are needle-phobic.

It's not like before, as we have one patient each to care for, and Covid-positive patients who have been vaccinated are doing well and have mild symptoms. They are mostly sick because of underlying health issues or they are elderly, over-weight, diabetic or frail. We transfer one man to the ward and another I extubate, as he is now breathing for himself and is recovering well. The third patient deteriorated and was trans-ferred to a more appropriate area. He has since died.

We spend hours where the air con doesn't work and the inside temperature is 32.9 degrees Celsius. The sweat trickles down your body so your scrubs are damp, and I am relieved I am wearing deodorant.

An old-fashioned air-con machine chunders away noisily, leaking water onto the floor. Its elephant-trunk-size tube goes up through a roughly cut hole in the ceiling – it achieves nothing. We are hot and tired, and we shout through the FFP3 masks above the noise of the air con. Why doesn't Pret sell ice cream?

My recently extubated patient was so hot, I manoeuvred his bed into the middle of the room, cables trailing, so the stream of almost-cool air from the outlet hit his feet. He made a kissing face at me and fell asleep. His feet may feel cooler but the thermometer is still recording a temperature more suited to a day on the beach. Our health and safety manual states no maxim temperature for staff to work in. We had to relocate a Covid area in order for the air con be repaired so that the temperature was more acceptable for patients and staff.

One of our nurses treated us to an iced coffee from Marks & Spencer.

*   *   *

We are yet to see the far-reaching consequences of Covid, but suicide among the young seems to be a regular occurrence and then there are those who delay coming into hospital because they are scared.

Tensions are high. There is enormous pressure to 'catch up', a daily race to find beds to keep the patient flow moving, from ED to the ward, to theatre, to Critical Care, back to the ward, then home. It's rarely smooth and this continuous coordination keeps our senior staff and bed managers permanently occupied. Any delay may block the next patient. There are always fewer beds than patients and never enough staff to manage these beds, though we may meet the minimum staffing criteria. It just takes one patient who, for whatever reason – unstable, confused, distressed, high body mass – requires the care of more than one nurse. It's never straightforward and each day is different, bringing new challenges.

Blue area closed, cleaned and re-opened three days later for two more Covid-positive patients, who are thankfully stable and doing well, and the air con is now fixed (as much as an ancient system can be fixed). Current temperature: 26 degrees Celsius – still beach-worthy, still sweaty, and so good to see some of our nurses sitting outside the pub drinking cold beer on my walk home.

Who knows if this is the early stages of a third wave. Time will tell.

*　　*　　*

I have received the following letter from Ray Symons, who was a patient on Covid ICU.

Dear Anthea,

I've been home from hospital now for just over a year, and I wanted to let you know that I am making a really good recovery and that you are one of the main reasons for that.

When I woke up from my coma, in St. George's, I was disorientated and uncertain. I found myself in a room on my own, unable to move or speak, and unable to see my wife or family. I was still having bad dreams and I was in quite a lot of pain. It was not entirely certain that I would survive. On reflection, it would have been easy for me to have become distressed and despondent and that would have made it more difficult for me to recover and rehabilitate. You did more than anyone to ensure that I didn't get down about things and remained engaged, optimistic and positive throughout.

You always made me feel very special. You took an interest in me and you paid attention to my little quirks, which might have seemed trivial at the time but were incredibly important to me. For example, you knew that I had developed a fixation for ice-cold drinks and food when I was unable to eat and receiving my food through a tube. So together with the other nurses you made sure that I had ice to suck on, even though you had to go up hill and down dale to find it. When, after a few weeks, my swallow was strong enough to allow me to eat for myself, you went out and got ice cream for me. I was really touched by that gesture.

On another occasion, you went to the shops and got a lovely birthday card for me to give to my wife and a bunch of flowers. I remember in my enfeebled state checking every half an hour or so that the card was still there on my bedside table. I waited until the last possible moment to write it so that my handwriting was as legible as possible.

You went far beyond the bounds of what might reasonably be expected from a carer when you arranged for me to see my wife on her birthday. What was most amazing was that by the time of her birthday, I had been transferred from ICU to a general ward in St. George's and so was no longer under your care. Nevertheless, you found time to come down to the general ward with a couple of colleagues, fix me up in a wheelchair and take me to see Jo in the garden. I remember that it was a rare rainy day in June, but for half an hour, while we were out in the garden, the clouds parted and we sat in the sunshine together. It was lovely. It was the first time we had been together in ten weeks.

It wasn't just me that you helped. You helped Jo as well. She was very anxious when I was in hospital, and that anxiety was increased by the rather intermittent contact she had with Kingston Hospital when I was there in a coma. She found communication with the ICU at St George's more predictable, which reduced her stress considerably. It was also lovely that you would arrange for me to be at the window in my room when Jo came up to St George's to bring snacks and treats for your team, so that I could wave to her in the courtyard. These little things made such a difference to my state of mind.

From where I was lying, it looked like nursing was a tough job, and I cannot imagine what the pressure and stress must have been like during that first wave last spring. It must have been hard enough just to keep up with core responsibilities. The fact that you did all of that and still found the time for so much extra kindness makes me feel very lucky and grateful to have been under your care. It sounds like a weird thing to say, but thanks to you and your colleagues I shall remember my time recovering in St George's with some fondness. It was not nice to be so ill, but it was lovely to be looked after by you.

Ray

19 July

Freedom Day.

It is time to move on, move forward. I have written these emails, kept this diary for almost 18 months, throughout the Covid Express journey that took us to a different time and place. My epistle began as an email to request cake and biscuits for the phenomenal yet broken and war-torn staff I have the very great honour of working alongside. I have observed, experienced and documented grief, laughter, horror, success, sadness, tragedy, strength, compassion and love – as well as sheer grit and determination, resilience and hope.

Critical Care nurses are superb human beings. Women and men from all over the world who have the skills, knowledge, expertise and capabilities to care for any injured or ill patient or medical emergency situation. These nurses have held up our world for months and months, and they will continue to do so, as that's what we do.

We have had the invaluable support from many places and people, those redeployed and removed from their usual place of work: nurses of all grades, doctors from all specialities, students, allied health professionals, volunteers, the army. Many people. It's the Critical Care nurses that 'carry the can'. Doctors prescribe and plan, but it is the nurses who deliver the day-to-day care and understand the nuances of caring for a sick and unstable patient.

We are the ones required to teach and lead and guide and support while doubling, trebling or quadrupling our workload, and always giving the best multi-organ support we can offer to our patients, despite the conditions, and while programming and operating complex machinery, pumps and monitors, and showing kindness and empathy to our patients and their family.

We help individuals transcend sickness or injury. We are instrumental in recovery, compassionate with death. We see the rawness of life. If you know a Critical Care nurse, salute them. We did this without being asked and without reward. We are tireless heroes.

I am so proud of my incredible crew and feel privileged to know them. We will fragment and disperse once this is all over, as they dismantle the different spaces. But the memories of the nurses that carried this catastrophe are now imprinted in the core of myself. There are no words to express my gratitude, respect and thanks to our nurses.

We are bold, powerful and beautiful, despite this monstrous world war that took over the life, touch and freedom of every single person. We rose up and fought back. We united as one powerhouse of endurance, and I feel honoured and proud to be a nurse. Covid restrictions took away our freedom, but my team came together, offering so much of themselves, working in parallel with the world.

*   *   *

A man was admitted with a spontaneous brain haemorrhage. A CT scan revealed this as unrecoverable. All his body could do was breathe; with ventilatory support providing oxygen his heart would continue to beat. The Critical Care consultant gently explained to the patient's devastated wife that there was nothing that could be done. Over the next few days she spent time with her husband and slowly accepted the horrendous fact that he would never return from this random insult from within his own body.

To further shatter this woman's world, a man arrived at the hospital and revealed himself to be the patient's lover. He had no intention of causing mental anguish; he was heartbroken to learn that the man he loved was dying. He shared the fact that for over 20 years the patient had led a double life. He had a wife and family he loved and adored, and he had a long-term male lover. The double life seemed to be born from the need to not hurt his family while remaining true to his sexual identity.

Over a few days, this inspirational, devastated wife learned, accepted and forgave, and when my patient died he was with the two people he loved most in the world. They were united in grief. The wife said, 'We have so much in common, as we both loved him.' I learned later that they became close friends.

This story, for me, demonstrates that love can transcend anything. Covid taught me so much about love, something I previously thought I knew and understood. Covid shattered our world but there is hope, and something powerful and beautiful will come out of this crisis.

We look to our recovery and to the future.

EPILOGUE

This is the end of this book but not the end of the story. Covid remains.

Covid ICU admissions are now driven by unvaccinated people. The virus is still here, looking to put its vicious claws into someone, anyone – regardless of age or skin colour or health status. It's like there is a new pandemic, a new variant.

'I can't do it again.' That is the mantra of our staff, and there is discomfort for us, caring for those who choose not to join the war to fight this enemy, an enemy that has divided people. Those who have their own personal reasons for being vaccinated or not, based on their individual understanding and rationale. Surely vaccines are our wall of defence?

So we plod on ... 10, 11, 14, 18 patients. Then someone dies and a few patients are discharged to the ward, and the numbers level out again. It's a low-level grumble in the background. Covid-positive patients who require Critical Care are admitted to our current Covid ICU. Our staff are battered, doing this yet again. Morale is low. It's not fair –

our precious nurses have to do this for a third time and again and again and again.

Covid-positive patients are blocking beds for the endless stream of backlogged elective surgery and ED admissions. Emergency cardiac admissions take whichever bed is free on our other units, as their space has been trumped by Covid.

I commented to a colleague about the amount of young people who have been admitted recently, who have suffered from an out of hospital cardiac arrest (OOHCA): a young mum out for a run, a man squeezing in a gym session after work and before meeting his friends for a beer. They now lie in our beds, attached to monitors and machines, while we gently explain to their devastated families that we have to wait and see how their hypoxic brain injury may affect their recovery and survival.

The reason so many of these patients are with us, my colleague pointed out, is that they have been relocated, as the unvaccinated claim the beds on our specialist cardiac ICU. We are trained to care for any patient requiring our care, so the patients are safe, but usually they would be housed within our cardiac unit.

It's impossible to get a GP appointment, and it takes longer for an ambulance to arrive – waiting times have increased exponentially. Discussing a rash over the phone with a stressed-out, overworked GP is not the excellence our health service strives for.

Forgetting is difficult but remembering is worse; I think everyone has been affected by this pandemic. Not just NHS staff, but everyone. This curse swerved no one. We need to return to normal. There are far-reaching consequences of Covid and some are invisible.

I watched a documentary about 9/11. The horror and shock, the legacy of living. Seeing and learning what the people on those planes and in the buildings that were struck must have experienced – choosing to jump from the Twin Towers rather than be burned alive – it's abhorrent.

I can identify with the feelings the firefighters experienced and how they are still affected 20 years later.

*　　*　　*

Lunch out, shared with close colleagues who are also my friends, I am bathed in Italian and Portuguese youthfulness. But we all still see demons and some spaces in our hospital induce anxiety and tachycardia. I do not know one single nurse who came out of this unscathed.

Data doesn't always tell the whole story about Covid. Statistics, numbers, news reports. The government estimates that in England approximately five million people aged 16 and over have not received the vaccine.

Multiple studies show coronavirus vaccines are highly effective in preventing serious illness, and side-effects are rare. Immunologists say even if you have had Covid, vaccination will boost your immunity further.

Some people are unable to be vaccinated due to medical reasons. The anti-vaccine reasons vary but people have a choice. Choice is good and democracy is important; however, their choice severely affects the rest of society. It affects the entire world as countries plod on, trying to vaccinate as many people as possible.

Nurses do not have a choice; we have to care for our patients regardless. Unless nurses leave for a different career, we care for any patient who comes through our doors.

We should move on now, let it go, learn to live with Covid. Choirs should sing, theatres perform; we need to meet people, drink Aperol, embrace our friends, shake hands, talk, share, laugh and live our lives, but above all ...

Love.

Love.

Love.

A massive thank you to our Covid heroes – NURSES.

ACKNOWLEDGEMENTS

In praise of love and biscuits …

I am indebted to the many people who have helped this book come about. Sophie, who coined its fabulous title, *Life, Death and Biscuits*, and who has provided years of rock-solid friendship through birth, death, breastfeeding, tears, hilarity and food; Nicola ('Nicky'), who's there for me 'when I'm not' and tolerates the crazy; Annette, who understands when it's not OK; my fantastic social media support team – Claudia, Ilaria, Agnese, Sophie, Paty, Paula and Mariyam – who are always consistent in their love and social media advice: 'You're beautiful.'

I am deeply grateful to James Steen, journalist, author, collaborator and friend, who listened, connected and understood. He supported me, shared Champagne, coffee, tears and poodles, 'tweaked' my story and turned it into a book.

Thank you to Charlie Brotherstone, who introduced me to the team at HarperCollins. They helped navigate me through the world of publishing, and my thanks go to my editors Kelly Ellis and Holly Blood, as well as Sarah Hammond (project editor), Steve Burdett (copy-editor), Holly Macdonald (cover designer), Liane Payne (picture researcher) and Alan Cracknell (production controller).

Pippa Harper, media manager at St George's, has been hugely helpful, and my thanks also goes to Jey Jeyanathan for his kindness, support and medical advice (and for always respecting nurses).

Thank you also to my surrogate 'children', who give so much every day and who inspired me to write that first email, and to my neighbours and local community, who supported and fed us, as well as to CriticalNhs, Empire Heroes and my 'stranger friend' Giles Sequeira, who is my fixer and main man.

Thanks especially to my patients – without them, life seems unimaginable.

In memory of Jonathan, my friend, my comfort, my beautiful tabby cat, 2016–2021.

A special thank you goes to those who showed me kindness, encouraged me, inspired me, stood by me, got drunk with me, comforted me, messaged me, worked with me, stayed late, understood, went the extra mile, gave me a lift and a place of safety, were flexible, were team players, and, most importantly, laughed and loved and cared with me: Aaron Madeira, Adriano Massari, Agnese Vitale, Agnieszka Crerar-Gilbert, Agnieszka Zajac, Aileen Concepcion, Aisling Burke, Alan Ducasse, Alan Millington, Alan Williams, Alexandra Kourompina, Alida Carrà, Alywin family, Amber Gray, Ambrosie Muchembled, Amelia Guyguyon, Amina Yusuf, Amy Fleming, Andy Harris, Angeline Degre, Angelika Kerlin, Angelo Almeida Rocha, Ann Bartrip, Ann Walker, Annabel Stratten, Annie Hammond, Amy McDonnell WASO, Anne Palmer, Annette McFadyen, Anton Trutor, Aoife Boyle, Aoife McCarthy, Argyro Zoumprouli, Arlene Domingo, Atif Mian, Atul Mehta, Becky Bryan, Belinda Bermudez, Beverley De Castro, Bhelyne Santos, Birds of Tokyo, Bridget Palmer, Bronwyn Hopper, Camilla Simpson, Carlotta Bianchi, Carmen Conçalves, Carmina Formantes-Aguirre, Caroline Davidson, Caroline Sharples, Cat Auld, Cat Pert, Cecile Dela Cruz, Charielyn Tamayo, Chloe Jones, Chris Blunden, Chris Brunker, Chris Ryan, Chris Smallwood, Claire Dalton, Claire Ostrowska, Coldplay, Cristina Ciuffreda, Claire Riddell, Clare Lucas, Claudia Gilbert-Allen, Clementina Olaniy, Connor Christie, Dagan Lonesdale, Daniela Barreiro, Dario Casserta, David Haughie, David Sterling, Debbie Swain, Demelza Jones, Diana Delgardo Lazo, Dolphine Masaki, Dominic Spray, Edel Neary, Edna Okyere, Elia Cappelletti, Elisabeth Watson, Elizabeth McFarlane, Ellie O'Connor, Emma D'Cruz, Empire Heroes, Empire Heroes community bakers, Faye Crathern, Flavia Di Bello, Francesca Robinson, Fraser Woolley, Fred Ahenkora, Full Fat cafe Balham, Gabor Zilahi, Gabrielle Blundell-Pound, Gabrielle Johnson, Garry Killick, Gary Grant, Gary Sanchez, Gavin Smith, Gemma Cohen, Gemma Fradin, Gemma Wallis, Georgia Petherick, Gianluca

Risolvo, Gihan Abuella, Giles Sequeira, Gillian Selman, Gillian Upton, Giorgia Imperoli, Grace Lacaden, Grace Okeke, Greg McAnulty, Halina Kerlin, Hannah Bishop, Happiness Amagboruju, Helen Farrah, Hina Ahmed, Hollmann Aya, Holly Cahill, Hornsby House School, Ilaria Bruno, Isa PereiraIsabelle Augier, Isabella Papp, Izzy Bohn, Izzy Walter, Jack Torrance, Jackie Williams, James Powys-Lybbe, James Steen, Jane Roe, Janice Barrett, Janneke Diemel, Jean-Philippe Blondet and team, Jen Tulloch, Jen Wetherden, Jenni Doman, Jenny James, Jerome Serwanga, Jessica Hackshaw, Jiji Manoj, Jo Cox, Jo Symons, Joanna Knowles, Joanne Lawson, John Allen, Jon Aron, Jonathan Ball, Jonathan Da Costa, Jonathan Silver, Jos Ewan, Jose Rio Mamon, Julia Reardon, Julian Roda Narro, Julie Noble, Karen Mheachair, Karin Falloon, Kat Somers, Kate Maleki, Kate Sankar, Kate Watson, Kate Woodhouse, Kathleen Dizon, Kathy Dalley, Katie Green, Keith Dicker, Keith Robertson, Kerry Smith, Kim Tatham, Kirsty Rae, Kirsty Yeong, Kitty Timpson, Kya O'Meara, Ladidne M'mem, Laine Magdaong, Lara Wyatt, Laura de la Pascua Marin, Laura Pender, Leane McCracken, Leaner Sequeira, Lesley Mclean, Liam Whitt, Linda Smith, Lindsey Izard, Ling Wong, Lisa Booker, Lisa French, Lisa Wrate, London scrubbers, Lorenzo Tiraboshi, Lou Eyeington, Louise Davey, Louise Stuart, Lucy Heywood, Maddy Sequeira, Manuel Aliano-Hermoso, Margo Watson, Maria Maiz Cordoba, Maria O'Riordan, Maria Thanasi, Mariam Davies, Marife Estrada, Mario Perera, Marivic Boeseta,

Mark Grimshaw, Mark Hamilton, Mark Russon, Mark Smith, Markus Vater, Maryiam Ba, Massimiliano Valcher, Matt Moore, Matthew Seligman, Maya Govender, Mayni Paul, Melissa Walton, Michael Canete, Mohammed Abedin, Mónica De La Fuente Izquierdo, Monica Ferrao, Morris Tolaram, Myrna Scott, Nana Frempomaa, Naomi Standard, Natasha Cardazzzone, Natasha Trenchard- Turner, Neil Howarth, Niall Barrett, Nick Herrtage, Nicola Fee, Nicola Small, Nicola Walker, Nikki Yun, Nirav Shah, Nyrina Barwise, Olly Blackford, Orsolya Miskolvi, Osvaldo Quadros, Parbatta Kunwar, Patricia Dowley, Patricia Thomas, Patry Espinoza, Paty Araujo, Paul Randall, Paul Silke, Paula Alves, Paula O'Shea, Paulo Castilho, Penny Mullord Stafford-Piper, Peter Gilbert-Allen, Peter Watson, Polly Downes, Polly Hitchcock, Punitha Gopinath, Rachael Harvey, Rachel Wood, Rafik Bedair, Ranjana KC, Raudzi Mandizvidza, Ray Symons, Rebecca Flanagan, Riccardo Malaspina, Richard Huie, Rizza Aban, Roah Khalid, Robin Dobinson, Romina Pepermans, Rory Scott, Rosalind Allen, Rutger Thiellier, Sacha Milroy, Sadik Alhassani, Sandra Micksch, Santiago Silva Parez, Sarà Ramos, Sarah Beeny, Sarah Farnell-Ward, Sarah Hales, Sarah Karslake, Sarah Millan, Sarah Pappalardo, Sarah Piper, Sarah Shoesmith, Sasha Brennan, Sasha Lewis, Shane Hopper, Shiela Mujer, Shreeja Dangol, Shrikresh Malde, Simon Leithhead, Sonia Forde at Body Potential, Sophie Jones, Sophie Nolloth, Sophie Ruston-Smith, Stacey Lane, Steph Ramsey, Stephen Ndoro, Steve Louis, Streatham & Clapham High School,

Susan Reynolds, Susannah Leaver, Suzanne Levy, Taina Pearson, Tammy Stracey, Tania Ferreira, Tessline Mathew, Tania Mariscal Lopez, Teareen Mamdeen, Titi Savanau, Toa Stappard, Toby Sullivan at Fit by Physio, Tooting Market, Tracey Campbell, Vanessa Elliot, Velinda Beran, Vicky Basini, Vicky Foroughi, Victoria Williams, Vilma Lewis and Yvette Skinner.

Thank you to the entire Critical Care team, to everyone who supported me through this journey and throughout the pandemic, my family, friends and colleagues. Laughter really is the best medicine. Love, laughter, life.

And never forget – Critical Care nurses are brilliant!

And I only asked for biscuits …